29.10.07

The philosophy of palliative care

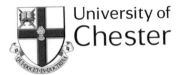
University of
Chester

This book is to be returned on or before the last date stamped below. Overdue charges will be incurred by the late return of books.

The philosophy of palliative care:critique and reconstruction

Fiona Randall
Consultant in Palliative Medicine
Royal Bournemouth and Christchurch Hospital Trust
Bournemouth, UK

R. S. Downie
Honorary Professorial Research Fellow
Emeritus Professor of Moral Philosophy
University of Glasgow
Glasgow, UK

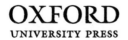

OXFORD
UNIVERSITY PRESS

OXFORD
UNIVERSITY PRESS

Great Clarendon Street, Oxford ox2 6DP

Oxford University Press is a department of the University of Oxford.
It furthers the University's objective of excellence in research, scholarship,
and education by publishing worldwide in

Oxford   New York

Auckland Cape Town Dar es Salaam Hong Kong Karachi
Kuala Lumpur Madrid Melbourne Mexico City Nairobi
New Delhi Shanghai Taipei Toronto

With offices in

Argentina Austria Brazil Chile Czech Republic France Greece
Guatemala Hungary Italy Japan South Korea Poland Portugal
Singapore Switzerland Thailand Turkey Ukraine Vietnam

Oxford is a registered trade mark of Oxford University Press
in the UK and in certain other countries

Published in the United States
by Oxford University Press Inc., New York

British Library Cataloguing in Publication Data
Data available

Library of Congress Cataloging in Publication Data
Randall, Fiona.
    The philosophy of palliative care: critique and reconstruction/Fiona Randall, Robin S. Downie.
    p. ; cm
Includes bibliographical references and index.
1. Palliative treatment–Philosophy. 2. Palliative treatment–Moral and ethical aspects.
[DNLM: 1. Palliative Care–ethics. 2. Philosophy, Medical. WB 310 R188p 2006] 1. Downie, R. S. (Robert
Silcock) 11. Title.
R726.8.R35 2006
616'.029–dc22

Typeset by SPI Publisher Services, Pondicherry, India
Printed in Great Britain
on acid-free paper by Biddles Ltd., King's Lynn

ISBN 0-19-856-736-7 (Pbk.: alk.paper)   978-0-19-856736-3 (Pbk.)

Foreword

David J. Roy

> *"Our unspoken assumptions have the force of revelation."*
> Seamus Heaney (1)

In palliative medicine and palliative care, the marshalling of knowledge, skills, and human presence to relieve pain, discomfort, nausea, fatigue, insomnia, anxiety, and many other kinds of distress also serves the deeper existential purpose of freeing up a sick and dying person's time. To free a gravely ill person's time of mind, memory, imagination, and feeling from the forces of agony that would compress that time into ever narrower black holes of suffering is palliative care's work of emancipation. The hope within that work is that personal time *freed from* the constrictions of distress will be *freed up for* experiences meaningful and powerful enough to demonstrate for persons, threatened with the loss of everything, "that for a short moment there is no death and time does not unreel like a skein of yarn thrown into an abyss" (2).

These lines from Czeslaw Milosz's poem, "Earth Again", are a symbol of the kinds of events and experiences that bring the *unconditioned* into people's lives. The *unconditioned* here refers to those unique experiences of grace, of gift, of word, of presence that can redeem tragedies of the past, fill a present threatened by absence and emptiness, and light a lamp in a future seemingly so short and dark.

The "Milosz Experiences" cannot be guaranteed, they cannot be measured or quantified, and the medical, nursing, and other allied palliative care professionals, as such, cannot deliver them. To think otherwise, to imagine that people professionally trained in palliative medicine and palliative care should, as an integral part of their competence, be able to bestow "Milosz Experiences" on suffering and dying people would be to submit these professionals and the persons in their care to unrealizable messianic expectations.

The Fiona Randall and Robin Downie critique and attempted reconstruction of the philosophy of palliative care directs a beam of critical reflection precisely onto such expectations and related assumptions in currently prevailing definitions, thinking, and writing about palliative care. The words of these writings, as the authors say, distil the philosophy and the philosophy directs the practice of palliative care, and the authors' prime concern is with the direction of this practice.

Our unspoken assumptions, to follow the poet, may well have the force of revelation. However, when these assumptions are spoken, the revelation may well be of how blind we have been or become. The assumptions enshrined in a philosophy of palliative care may well—if they are *both* unquestioned and unexamined *and* persistently repeated and amplified—blind us to what we should not be doing, and are continuing to do; may blind us also to what we should be doing, and are failing to do. This Fiona Randall and Robin Downie critique of the philosophy of palliative care may, I think, help us all to look once again at ideas to which we may have become blind.

If authors can fail in their writing of a book, readers can also fail in their reading of it. A book attempting to unmask the mismatches between the rhetoric and realities of palliative care would fail, I think, if it did not arouse moments of indignation and astonishment in some, if not all, of its readers. We do tend to get a bit touchy when ideas dear to us are brought into question, and this book, I think, will not fail to bring into question some ideas many of us have long cherished about palliative care.

Readers, however, will fail in their reading of this book if they become frozen in one or another of their moments of indignation, astonishment or shock over what they are reading. The deep pitfall to be avoided would be the failure to enter into the critique, and to engage that critique actively, from beginning to end. Engaging a critique carries the freedom to disagree, a freedom for reasoned disagreement that explains itself.

Readers could also fail in their reading of this book if they would allow a moment of indignation or profound disagreement to convince them that the authors are setting out to dismantle palliative care. Indeed, these authors are doing exactly the contrary. They are writing their critique out of a belief and conviction "that palliative care has an expanding future at the heart of health care". That is why they are so involved in examining the assumptions currently governing thinking, research, and practice in palliative care.

In their thinking about the problems in the world of palliative care, Fiona Randall and Robin Downie, it would seem to me, are illustrating the power of Albert Einstein's approach to problems in the world at large: "The problems that exist in the world today cannot be solved by the level of thinking that created them" (3).

References

1) Heaney S. *The Haw Lantern*. London, Boston: Faber and Faber, 1987: 19.

2) Milosz C. *Unattainable Earth*. Translated by the author and Robert Hass. New York: The Ecco Press, 1968: 8.

3) Einstein, A. Einstein's Aphorisms. Minds and Mental Matters.
http://www.websophia.com/faces/einstein.html (accessed on October 12, 2005)

Preface

The practice of palliative care goes back to the hospices of the Middle Ages. Out of these there emerged a philosophy of 'a good death', which was developed in a broader way in the twentieth century by Dame Cicely Saunders and expressed in her many writings and lectures. The core element of this philosophy was an emphasis on the primacy of the personal, of the needs and wishes of the individual patient, in the context of the increasingly impersonal nature of modern technological medicine.

More recently the insights of Dame Cicely have been condensed into a definition of palliative care by the World Health Organization (WHO). This definition, with its expansion in writings by the WHO and many others, has become so influential that it is widely seen as constituting a distinctive approach to end-of-life care—the 'palliative care approach'. The 'palliative care approach' was originally adopted with cancer patients, but there is currently a move in many countries to extend it to all end-of-life situations. Indeed, in the UK the highly influential National Institute for Clinical Excellence (NICE) goes even further and suggests that the 'palliative care approach' should be the model for care at all stages of a disease.

Now, in view of this move to make the 'palliative care approach' the model for care in all areas and at all stages of an illness, it is important to pause and review the approach, to consider the evidence for its effectiveness. After all, if the 'palliative care approach' is truly a philosophy of patient care, and indeed one which is claimed to be superior to other philosophies of patient care, then, like all philosophies, it should be open to a critique which investigates what it means, its internal consistency, the evidence for its effectiveness, and in general its strengths and weaknesses. We shall argue that it has significant weaknesses.

We must however stress that we are by no means intending to suggest that the palliative care approach should be entirely rejected—far from it. But it will be our argument that palliative care has become over-professionalized, too precious, and too busy. We shall recommend a return to a simpler approach to patient care at the end of life. Palliative care philosophy was developed partly as a reaction against over-zealous medical interventions at the end of life. But similarly, the assessments, questionnaires, counselling, and measurement scales, which have become so typical of the palliative care approach, can also be seen as a kind of harassment at the end of life. Indeed, the popularity of the term 'assessment tool' is all too indicative of the fact that professional engineering is replacing quiet listening. At the very least the evidence for the effectiveness of such procedures requires scrutiny.

In developing our argument we shall begin by examining the roots of palliative care, its conceptual framework, and its distinctive contribution (Part 1). We shall then suggest that this distinctive identity is being lost or distorted; care which should be expressed from inside a human relationship is becoming an externally imposed intervention based on professional assessments. To provide detailed illustrations of these criticisms we review the central concepts of palliative care philosophy: quality of life, autonomy, dignity, patient-centredness, and the priority assigned to relatives in the remit of care. Such concepts are all part of the common currency of palliative care, but their immediate appeal means that it is easy to lose sight of the moral problems implicit in their practical implementation. The main palliative care interventions are symptom-control and emotional, psychological, and spiritual care. We go on to discuss these and also the difficulties in cardio-pulmonary resuscitation (CPR), and advance statements as they affect palliative care (Part 2). All health care policies have resource implications and at the end of Part 2 we discuss these in the palliative care approach, as defined in the WHO statement.

We use the current (third) edition of the Oxford Textbook of Palliative Medicine (OTPM) as our main resource. This has three advantages from our point of view. Firstly, it provides us with a recent, detailed, and comprehensive summary of what is considered to be best practice in the specialty. Secondly, since it is extensively referenced, it has been unnecessary to repeat the references in our text. Thirdly, it is the reference textbook which we considered was most likely to be accessible to readers of this book. Our book should be considered as a reflective (and sometimes critical) commentary on the moral assumptions of what is considered best practice. We shall draw attention to the inflated and often contradictory claims made in the literature of palliative care—its rhetoric—and seek to defend its clinical practice—its enduring reality.

In our reconstruction of the philosophy of palliative care we shall make positive suggestions in the course of each chapter, and finally we shall draw these suggestions together and outline a framework for the reconstruction of the philosophy of palliative care (Part 3). Basically we shall suggest that if palliative care is to evolve and influence other areas of health care it should shed some of its professional complexities. In its original simplicity it appealed to the humanity which was being lost in the measurements and technology of modern medical practice. If it can reconsider the usefulness of its own measurements and complexities it can still have that appeal.

No one can fail to be impressed by the dedication of the actual practitioners of palliative care—the professionals and the many lay helpers. Our critique is directed not at them but at the confused philosophy which cannot, in reality, be enacted in clinical practice. Yet it is possible to construct a coherent philosophy of palliative care which defines desirable and achievable aims for patients, professionals, and families. We attempt to do this, and offer this book as a contribution to the reconstruction of the philosophy of palliative care.

Fiona Randall, Royal Bournemouth and Christchurch Hospital Trust
R. S. Downie, University of Glasgow
Spring 2005

Acknowledgments

We would like to thank Dr David Roy for taking time from his busy life as Editor of the *Journal of Palliative Care* to write a Foreword. His editorials sometimes celebrate views which are controversial or critical of received opinion, so we thought he would not reject out of hand our radical critique and reconstruction of the philosophy of palliative care. To say this is not of course to suggest that Dr Roy would endorse all or any of our proposals. But we are very grateful for his interest.

We must thank our colleagues for their forbearance while the book was being researched and written: they were very patient. More than that, they were the inspiration which set us going to investigate the discrepancy between the ambitions of the palliative care philosophy to invade all aspects of the lives of patients and their families and the common sense approach we find in actual practice. The purpose of a philosophy of palliative care is to guide practice. It was from the generous acceptance and good humour of our patients and their families that we have learned the philosophy offered in this book. We are therefore above all grateful to our patients.

F.R.
R.S.D.

Contents

List of abbreviations

A&E	Accident and Emergency
BMA	British Medical Association
BMJ	*British Medical Journal*
CPR	Cardio-pulmonary resuscitation
GMC	General Medical Council
GP	General Practitioner
HRQL	Health Related Quality of Life
JPC	*Journal of Palliative Care*
NICE	National Institute for Clinical Excellence
NHS	National Health Service
OTPM	*Oxford Textbook of Palliative Medicine* (3rd edn unless otherwise specified)
QALY	Quality Adjusted Life Year
WHO	World Health Organization

Part 1

Framework and concepts

Roots, traditions, and philosophy

Introduction and aims

In an editorial in the *Journal of Palliative Care* David J. Roy speaks with strong approval of certain views of the 1981 Nobel Laureate for literature, Elias Canetti. David Roy approves of his views because 'Canetti was able to say wild, impossible, unheard of things about death because he was able—a supreme freedom—to think thoughts others dared not imagine'.[1]

Paradoxically, in the very same edition of the journal we learn that Ruth Macklin was the subject of much angry protest for her article in the *British Medical Journal* (*BMJ*) entitled 'Dignity is a useless concept'.[2] Now it is true that the title is a trifle provocative, but Ruth Macklin presents us with an argued point of view in saying 'wild, impossible, unheard of things'. Why then should she have attracted such an onslaught? We shall later return to the concept of dignity and discuss it in some detail, but we mention the case of Ruth Macklin here because it draws attention to the daunting task ahead of us when we attempt to offer a critique of the philosophy of palliative care. Our hope is that we can encourage those in palliative care to follow us and think 'thoughts that others dared not imagine'. The 'thought' in question is that, as well as its celebrated strong points and unique insights, palliative care does have considerable weaknesses in its philosophy and in its approaches to patient care. It will be our contention that aspects of the philosophy of palliative should be modified or sometimes totally abandoned.

We are well aware that none of us likes our cherished beliefs and practices to be challenged, and of course there may be adequate replies to some of our criticisms. Nevertheless, our hope is that those who are committed to the care of the terminally ill may be willing to consider whether that care and commitment is always well-directed.

Of course, it is easier to offer criticisms than constructive suggestions, but we shall try to avoid being simply negative. We hope to make positive suggestions for the future of palliative care in the twenty-first century.

Indeed, a large portion of this book will be devoted to offering some positive ideas.

It follows, then, that our overall aim in this study is to suggest directions in which palliative care should evolve while retaining its essence as a distinctive specialty. The pursuit of this aim requires a critique of the philosophy of palliative care as it is laid down in the World Health Organization's (WHO) definition. In order to be fair to the WHO and to enable readers to refer to it, we will quote in full the definition and its supplementary detail as written in 2002.

> Palliative care is an approach that improves the quality of life of patients and their families facing the problems associated with life-threatening illness, through the prevention and relief of suffering by means of early identification and impeccable assessment and treatment of pain and other problems, physical, psychosocial and spiritual.

As a further explanation, the WHO develops the points in the definition as follows:

> Palliative care provides relief from pain and other distressing symptoms, affirms life and regards dying as a normal process, and intends neither to hasten nor to prolong death. Palliative care integrates the psychological and spiritual aspects of patient care, and offers a support system to help patients live as actively as possible until death. It also offers a support system to help the family cope during the patient's illness and in their own bereavement. Using a team approach, palliative care addresses the needs of patients and their families, including bereavement counselling if necessary. It enhances quality of life, and may positively influence the course of the illness. It is applicable early in the course of the illness with other therapies that are intended to prolong life, such as chemotherapy or radiation therapy, and includes those investigations needed to better understand and manage distressing clinical complications.[3]

The general strategy of the book will be to begin each chapter with an exposition and critique of a given aspect of palliative care, as described above, and then to go on to suggest possible lines for its future reconstruction. We must stress that we are not primarily criticizing the wording of the WHO definition. The words of the definition express deeply-rooted attitudes which palliative care professionals adopt and which determine their practice; the words distil the philosophy and the philosophy directs the practice. Our concern is with the direction of that practice.

This book is written in the belief that palliative care has an expanding future at the heart of health care, and that it has the potential to influence for the better other areas of health care. But in order to do this, it must first reconsider some of its cherished beliefs. Hence, we hold that there is a need for a critique of the philosophy of palliative care to make room for fresh growth.

As we said, this philosophy is expressed in practice, especially as staff often work in specialist units (sometimes called hospices) set apart from the mainstream of health care. Our questioning of this philosophy has arisen directly out of clinical experience, both in such a specialist unit and also in general hospital and primary care settings. In addition to this practical experience, participation in general professional ethics committees and in the teaching of health care ethics to professionals in other specialties has encouraged us to examine specialist palliative care from other perspectives.

When critics make suggestions about possible improvements to existing practices there is often despondency among practitioners, for such improvements usually involve extra activities, new safeguards, or new aspects of care. Our suggestions however do not involve new complexities in practice. On the contrary, we shall criticize the practice of palliative care for becoming too elaborate, too intrusive, too precious. What we shall recommend is a return to the original simplicity of palliative care and its philosophy as it was first formulated in the twentieth century by Dame Cicely Saunders.

We are now in a position to be able to state the aims of this study. These are:

- Part 1: In this Section we discuss the general philosophical framework including its roots and tradition, and indicate the main lines of our critique. We consider, critically, the central concepts of palliative care: quality of life; dignity, autonomy, rights, and human rights; and the priority assigned to relatives in the remit of care.
- Part 2: Here we shall discuss critically the main types of intervention in palliative care, such as symptom-control and life-prolonging treatment; resuscitation and advance statements; psychosocial and spiritual care; and the resource implications of these.
- Part 3: This Section pulls together the positive suggestions of previous chapters and builds on them to reconstruct a positive philosophy for the future of palliative care.

1.1 Roots and traditions

The roots of modern palliative care are of course to be found in religious orders concerned with the care of the dying. These orders had a conception of a 'good death', which involved an acceptance of human mortality and a recognition that human weakness and sin could be forgiven, and that death itself could be seen as the signature of a meaningful life. Moreover, death was seen in an earlier age to be a family or community event, rather than a medical event. Relatives and friends would be with the dying, offering support and comforting each other.

Such ideas passed into the twentieth century hospice movement and can be seen in operation in hospices such as St Joseph's or St Christopher's. Concepts such as 'meaning', 'fulfilment', or 'authenticity' became the substitutes for religious conceptions, and family involvement took the form of encouragement to relatives to visit the patient whenever possible (unlike the restricted visiting hours typical in the 1960s of mainstream hospitals). Religious ideas that each person is uniquely loved as the child of God, became secularized in ideals such as 'you matter because you are you'.[4]

In addition to the religious background to twentieth century hospice thinking there was another influential strand in its development. This strand expressed a reaction against excessive use of medical technology. The second half of the twentieth century was of course the period in which there were spectacular advances in medical technology, both in pharmaceuticals and in surgery. The medical profession, and indeed the general public, were rightly impressed with these advances which resulted in new ways of prolonging life. Sometimes these life-prolonging measures were justifiable, but those in the new hospice movement often believed that what was being prolonged was simply the process of dying. Hence, in addition to the ideas of acceptance, meaning, and fulfilment, we find a second strand in the modern hospice movement expressed in new concepts such as 'dignity' and 'quality of life'. This strand in hospice thinking was expressed by saying that patients did not enter a hospice to die, but rather to live until they died; and that what mattered was not quantity, but quality of life.

We might sum this up, admittedly in an over-simplified way, by saying that in the period 1960–80 hospices had developed a philosophy which separated them from mainstream medicine. They were often separate physically from mainstream hospitals, and their approach to the treatment of the terminally ill was radically different. For mainstream medicine, death was a medical failure. Diseases had always to be 'fought', patients had to be resuscitated and snatched back from the 'Enemy', and white-coated doctors appeared as heroes in the new phenomenon of the medical 'soap opera'. For the small minority who adhered to a hospice philosophy, death was something which had to be accepted and could be meaningful. The mainstream idea of 'curing' was replaced in the hospice movement with the older idea of 'healing'. Indeed, it should be noted that the word 'healing' comes from the Anglo-Saxon word 'haelan' meaning 'to make whole'. Hence, 'whole person care' or 'holistic care' became terms of hospice philosophy. What we have appearing from the 1960s are two different ways of looking at health care.

1.2 **Two traditions of health care**

It would be quite wrong to describe these as new ways of looking at health care. In fact, both go back to the origins of Western medicine in the Greek world. It is important for us to say a little more about these two traditions because the ideas which each expresses are central to our critique and positive suggestions. We must of course stress that the origins of medicine are obscure and their scholarly complexities are irrelevant to our theme. In identifying the two traditions of medicine we are concerned with two tendencies in medical practice, rather than historical detail, even if that detail were available. These tendencies were present at the very beginning of Western medicine and we shall discuss them in terms of the two traditions.

The first tradition is that of Hippocrates, and that is the tradition which is dominant at the moment. Hippocrates was a Greek physician who was born around 460 B.C. He and his School were dedicated to investigating the rational, scientific basis of medicine. This scientific approach ignores the individuality of patients and instead concentrates on what diseases have in common. It is assumed that diseases follow a pattern, the causal laws of which can be discovered. When they are discovered, treatments may be devised and applied regardless of the individual experience of illness and disease. The central doctrine of the Hippocratic school is that every disease, every human ailment, has a cause which can be discovered and is curable, and that this knowledge is generalizable. This belief is the foundation of Western scientific medicine, and continues to inspire research and treatment.

The second tradition of medicine is also Greek in origin and is older than the Hippocratic tradition, although both flourished together. It is that of Asklepius. Asklepius is a shadowy figure in Greek thought. He was believed to be the son of the god Apollo (the god of healing and the arts) by a mortal woman. The Asklepian tradition stresses healing, but in the context of our acceptance of our mortality. Patients who sought healing at the temples of Asklepius tended to be those who were incurable by the practical means known at the time. Nevertheless, they sought relief from their suffering. The temples of Asklepius, which were the centres of healing, contained harmless serpents (*coluber longissima*). It was thought to be the mystical hypnotic gaze of the serpent which was healing and the fact that serpents change their skin was also symbolic. Moreover, the atmosphere of the temple and the quiet repose and dreams of the patients were important in the healing process, for the healing comes from within the patient. There is an important contrast here with the Hippocratic tradition of modern medicine where the emphasis is on external intervention.

The Asklepian tradition, of the healing gaze of the serpent and the changes coming from within the patient (as in changing one's skin), translates well into palliative care. In a sense the gaze corresponds to the doctor's attention to the patient, to the careful waiting and listening, and to acceptance of this patient as a unique and important person in the context of our knowledge of our humanity. Holistic care, when seen in this way, is unobtrusive to the patient's personality and privacy, does not threaten their integrity, and is not manipulative. Healing derives from the careful application of our knowledge while constantly attending to the patient.

Perhaps we may introduce here an analogy we shall develop in our final chapter—between medicine and fine art. Dr Marie Therese Southgate, who was Deputy Editor of the *Journal of the American Medical Association*, writes of the similarities between the artist and the physician. Both have a common goal—to complete what nature cannot bring to a close. She argues that this is done by paying attention: 'The physician attends the patient; the artist attends nature. If we are attentive in looking, in listening and in waiting, then sooner or later something in the depths of ourselves will respond'.[5]

The Greeks followed both traditions concurrently. Patients would go to physicians who followed the Hippocratic tradition of rational treatment. The skills of the physician were practised, but if they failed to bring healing the patient would pursue the Asklepian method. The physicians of the Hippocratic tradition respected and welcomed the Asklepian tradition. Patients benefited from both approaches to healing.

In modern health care, the Hippocratic tradition certainly has the upper hand: evidence-based medicine is dominant in all spheres. Doctors are increasingly exhorted to follow protocols, guidelines, and patient pathways. Palliative care has embraced this culture too. There are many life-prolonging and symptom control treatments now available in palliative medicine and these may well be used in the best interests of patients. But palliative care must also retain the Asklepian tradition, which stresses the attention which should be given to each patient with their story, and their own values. 'Quality of life', 'dignity', 'meaningfulness', 'holistic care', even 'spirituality', are as vibrant in palliative care now as they ever were in the hospices of an earlier age. Indeed, the authors of the chapter on 'Quality of life' in the *Oxford Textbook of Palliative Medicine*, 3rd edn (*OTPM*) note that while in the period 1961–65 there were no papers at all indexed under 'quality of life' in Medline, by 1996–2000 there were an astonishing 12,749![6]

Yet this proliferation of papers, on what has become one of the central concepts of palliative care, is a symptom of what we shall diagnose as a serious disease in the palliative care approach. The disease is characterized by the invasion of the central and distinctive concepts of palliative care—those characteristic of the Asklepian tradition—by methods and interpretations characteristic of the Hippocratic tradition. The acceptance of our mortality, the idea of peace at the last, and connected ideas, have been medicalized and associated with training courses and measurable outcomes. The expression 'quality of life'—innocuous enough in itself in ordinary conversation—has become a piece of medical jargon giving rise to an enormous literature on questionnaires, scales, and numbers. The natural sadness which accompanies the end of a life, and the sorrow of friends and family, have become medical conditions requiring assessment and treatment. Again, some patients in their last weeks may wish to review their lives or relationships, but others may not. Yet the doctrine is that they should all be encouraged or 'counselled' to talk about their lives and relationships. The idea that death is a matter concerning the whole family has become a doctrine that relatives are as much objects of palliative care concern as the actual patients. To sum this up, the Asklepian tradition has become distorted because it is being interpreted in terms of the protocols, training courses, questionnaires, scales, and measurements which have become dominant in the Hippocratic tradition at the present time. Our critique will be directed at this distortion.

1.3 **Consumerism in health care**

In addition to the distortion of the simple Asklepian ideas of the early hospice movement, there is another current of contemporary western culture which has profoundly affected palliative medicine, indeed, health care as a whole. That is what we may term 'consumerism', or more generally, a rights-based individualism.

In developing this point we should first note that the doctrine of consent to treatment entered health care originally as a common law idea—that non-consensual touching is a criminal offence. Hence, patients must give their consent to examination and subsequent treatment. It follows from this doctrine that an informed and competent patient's refusal of treatment, even of life-saving treatment, is always legally valid and binding on doctors. This accepted doctrine of common law was increasingly interpreted from the 1970s in terms of a misunderstanding of the philosopher Kant's doctrine of the 'autonomy of the will'. We shall devote a chapter to this important confusion so will confine ourselves here to noting that by 'autonomy' Kant meant the ability we have to stand back from our own desires and act in terms of rules valid for all, or to be impartial.

The doctrine has however been given a consumerist interpretation and has come to mean in health care ethics that patients are entitled or have the right to be given the treatments they want. This is often called 'patient self-determination' or 'patient choice'. Indeed, as we shall see, some commentators claim that respecting patients' dignity requires giving them what they want, handing out the medical treatments they choose, even if the medical view is that what they want or choose is not in their best interests. In other words, the simple hospice view that 'you matter because you are you' has come to mean that you should be given the treatments you want. This, as we shall later argue, is a confused doctrine which has distorted treatments in palliative care and more widely.

We have discussed the roots and traditions of palliative care and current influences on its philosophy, and have given hints on the directions which our critique might take. But we have not so far explained in any detail the sense in which we shall use the term 'critique', and more importantly the sense in which there is a 'philosophy' of palliative care in the first place. Let us begin with the easier task of explaining what we mean by a 'critique'.

1.4 Critique

We are using the term 'critique' in the sense of the philosopher Immanuel Kant, when he speaks, for example, of a 'critique of pure reason'. His critique of pure reason consists in his attempt to establish the limits of pure reason. He is obviously not dismissing the whole concept but is investigating it with the aim of discovering what can and cannot be established by pure reason. In a similar way we are not rejecting the whole idea of a philosophy of palliative care but attempting to establish the strong and weak points of the current WHO philosophy. This is particularly important in view of the facts mentioned earlier: that those working in palliative care characteristically see themselves as different from other health care practitioners, and that they often work in locations which are physically separate from both primary and secondary health care. Our 'critique', then, will not be entirely a negative affair, but rather it will involve looking at some of the central ideas of palliative care from the perspective of colleagues in other health care disciplines.

Let us turn now to the idea of a 'philosophy' of palliative care. Two questions arise immediately. Firstly, we ask whether the WHO is really expressing a 'philosophy' at all (Section 1.5), and secondly, we ask what it is that this statement is striving to achieve (Section 1.6).

1.5 A 'philosophy' of palliative care

It might be objected that the WHO is not offering a 'philosophy' of palliative care at all but simply a definition. But what kind of definition is it? It is certainly much more than a dictionary definition. The *Oxford English*

Dictionary (*OED*) reports that (from 1588) the verb 'to palliate' means 'to alleviate the symptoms of a disease, to mitigate the sufferings of, to ease'. It would follow that palliative care is simply the branch of health care concerned with that activity, just as orthopaedics is the branch concerned with correcting injuries and deformities of bones. The *OED* is simply reporting how the words 'palliative' or 'to palliate' are used in ordinary speech. The WHO is clearly going well beyond this. Let us compare the 'definition' of 'health' offered by the WHO in 1946: 'Health is a state of complete physical, mental and social well-being, and not merely the absence of disease or infirmity'.[7]

This definition has several characteristics. Firstly, it is not reporting how the word 'health' is used; rather it is attempting to say something about the thing itself—health. Secondly, it is attempting to persuade us to see health in a much wider way than at that period had been common (i.e. involving the social and psychological). Thirdly, it was intended to influence health care practice; or, in other words, it had a normative function. To say all this, however, is tantamount to saying that the WHO definition of health was introducing, via a persuasive definition of health, a philosophy of health promotion.

All the above characteristics hold of the WHO 'definition' of palliative care: it is not reporting word usage; it is saying something about the activity of palliative care; and it is intended to influence practice. In short, the WHO definition is really the condensation of a 'philosophy'. But what sense of 'philosophy' is involved? Let us look at typical descriptions of 'philosophy'.

Philosophy itself cannot be easily or simply defined, but one view is that its main purpose is the critical examination of assumptions and arguments. A critical evaluation characteristic of philosophy begins as a critique of assumptions which then goes on to a critique of argument. It is in this sense of philosophy that we shall offer a critique of palliative care. On the other hand, the WHO statement of the philosophy of palliative care is certainly not a critical evaluation of assumptions, but instead is more like a list of assumptions. Nothing in the statement encourages questioning of those assumptions. It seems that the statement is not really 'philosophical' in this sense at all, although perhaps it is related to philosophy in the sense that it is at least a list of assumptions.

Carl Elliott, a doctor and a philosopher, in describing what he calls the 'traditional conception' of philosophy, provides us with a second account of philosophy. He notes that 'the aim of philosophy is to provide us with general explanations of the way things are, and ultimate justifications for our ethical and epistemological practices'.[8] The WHO statement does not explain the way things are in relation to palliative care, although it might perhaps be making a statement about the way it thinks things ought to be. Furthermore, it certainly does not provide us with any justification, ultimate or otherwise, for those assumptions so it is not a philosophy statement in the traditional sense either.

There is a third, a non-professional, sense of 'philosophy'. This is found in claims such as 'My philosophy, or my philosophy of life, is. . . .' followed by a list of beliefs about what I ought to do, and my attitudes to others and so on. This sense of 'philosophy' is close to the idea of an ideology, since it is a statement of assumptions, beliefs, or values held by a group of people, in this case by the WHO representing health care professionals who specialize in palliative care.

This sense of 'philosophy' resembles a statement of a religious faith. Firstly, it is similar in that no grounds for the assertions it makes are given, and indeed it may not be possible to prove the assertions in the way that statements of fact can be proven. Secondly, its assertions are thought to express truths which are self-evident to professionals working in the field. Thirdly, like a faith, those truths are not self-evident to all people, for it is clear that many professionals working outside the context of specialist palliative care might not accept or follow the normative content of the statement. For example, they would not consider that the relatives should form part of the remit of care. Fourthly, its critics may be viewed as a threat, or perhaps are to be pitied, since they are unable to accept the truths self-evident to others. Lastly, it resembles a faith in that its articles declare not just what one ought to believe but how one ought to live.

Supporters of the WHO statement might object that this interpretation is unfair. They may claim that it is not strictly a statement of faith, rather it presents a reasoned point of view, and in being a reasoned point of view it is more like a philosophy in the traditional sense. They may argue that there is evidence from clinical practice to support the set of beliefs it describes. They might further state that commitment to this set of beliefs follows from general beliefs in the importance of close relationships and of psychological as well as physical well-being. But if it is indeed a reasoned point of view then it should be open to a critique. Such a critique would examine its assumptions and any arguments supporting them. Palliative care does not have such a critique, but we aim to offer one in this book, and follow it with an attempt at a reasoned statement of how the philosophy be reconstructed. We shall continue to speak of the 'philosophy' of palliative care as laid down by the WHO, but it must always be remembered that the WHO statement is simply the expression of a set of beliefs rather than a reasoned point of view.

1.6 The normative function of a philosophy of palliative care

At the end of Section 1.4 we raised two questions: whether the WHO is really expressing a philosophy, and what it is that the WHO is trying to achieve by their statement. In answer to the first question we have suggested that it is a philosophy, but only in the minimum sense of 'my philosophy' i.e. a set of beliefs, not necessarily reasoned to any convincing extent. It is now possible to address the second question—namely, what the explicit statement of the 'philosophy' is aiming to achieve. It seems that its function is not simply to state what palliative care is about, by way of a description of the way things are, but rather to fulfil a normative function in stating the way things ought to be. It is a statement about how health care professionals ought to care for people whose illness is incurable and progressive to the point of death. Now a statement about how health care professionals ought to care for people as they approach death can take us along two different paths, which we shall call the 'theoretical' and the 'practical'. These terms must not be taken to be mutually exclusive for, as we shall see, the theoretical can have practical implications, and the practical makes theoretical assumptions; the paths can overlap. We shall now investigate where each path is leading.

1.7 **Theoretical questions**

Since the philosophy proposed relates to care at the end of life and implies acceptance of our mortality, then any discussion about palliative care occurs against the background of those major questions which relate to the meaning of life and death, or what constitutes a good life (and perhaps death) for a person. The answers to such questions are what traditional philosophy calls 'ultimate justifications' for our actions, or ultimate explanations of what we think is right. The WHO philosophy of palliative care does not contain explicit statements about the meaning of life or what constitutes a good life for a person. Yet it is intended to influence, and does influence, the way professionals care for patients at the end of life. In so doing, it implies that there is a 'right way of living and dying' for both patients and professionals. But the 'right way of living and dying' must depend on answers to the ultimate questions about what makes life worthwhile and about the meaning of life. It is perhaps strange that the philosophy describes the right way of living and dying in the context of palliative care without even alluding to those ultimate questions or providing any answers to them. The explanation may be that the origins of palliative care philosophy are religious, but the practitioners wish their special type of care to be widely available so they do not make explicit the metaphysical beliefs on which the philosophy is based.

It is not just in the sphere of palliative care that the ultimate questions are not acknowledged or addressed. Carl Elliott comments that 'Bioethics assumes it is about conduct and character, or, more narrowly, human obligations to each other', but that it does not ask or answer the ultimate questions about the meaning of life.[9] Instead, it asks only indirectly and unsatisfactorily (via the 'quality of life' concept), what makes life worth living. He goes on to ask 'Is it possible to think philosophically about the sense of life, and how it is situated in relation to other lives and to the institutions of medicine, once we have given up on ultimate explanations?'.[10] This is an important question, for the background philosophies of palliative care and of bioethics are each attempting to influence people into the 'right way of living and dying' without making explicit the answers and explanations which must act as reasons why one life or death should be better than any other life or death. It is not reasonable for the philosophy of palliative care, and for bioethics in general, to try to influence people into living life in a particular way without basing the values and assumptions put forward on answers to the ultimate questions. We shall later propose some answers or at least, more modestly, some ways of approaching the ultimate questions (Chapter 9).

We have argued that some answers to ultimate questions are called for if one is in the end to justify attempts to influence ways in which other people live and die at the ends of their lives. We suggested that palliative care, no less than other specialties, assumes answers to these questions but without any explicit defence or justification. Although we called this the 'theoretical' aspect of the WHO philosophy statement, it obviously has important practical implications. But there is another aspect of palliative care which has practical implications and that is the ethical aspect. Perhaps more than any other health care discipline palliative care raises ethical problems. We shall go on to suggest a way of tackling such problems in the next Section.

1.8 **Practical questions: ethics**

As an introduction to this discussion we should note that the approach to ethical questions in palliative care is open to criticism in that it is too much based on generalizations, such as that the patient's autonomy must always be respected. Such distortions are the ethical analogue of blind obedience to the claims of evidence-based medicine and the protocols based on it. Rules, generalizations and broad principles have their place in the search for humane decisions in ethics. But we must always come down to the individual case. A portion of our positive suggestions for the evolution of palliative care involves a development of this case-based approach to ethical decision-making.

We have both frequently been asked, together and separately, to speak at conferences and other meetings devoted to health care ethics. Sometimes the topics are specific, such as the rights and wrongs of advance statements, but it is our experience that at any ethics conference someone will be invited to speak about a 'framework' or a 'foundation' for ethical decision-making. Such a framework is often described as an 'ethical theory', from which, it is hoped, principles and rules can be derived to govern individual actions. For example, Childress and Beauchamp in their influential work *Principles of biomedical ethics* proposed four principles which, even though not fully grounded in a comprehensive theory, were said to be sufficient as a framework for describing ethical problems and reaching solutions.[11] They discussed at some length the characteristics of an ideal ethical theory, but noted that to date no single theory had satisfied them all.

Daniel Callahan, in describing the impact of ethical theory in the development of bioethics, states that 'Good ethical theory, it was believed, should be objective, rational, internally coherent and consistent, universally applicable, detached from individual self-interest, and impersonal in its capacity to transcend the particularities of time and culture'. He suggests that one might be able to frame a logically consistent moral theory, but 'the hard part is to devise a theory that can readily join universality and the moral complexity of everyday life. A flavor of cruel fanaticism seems often to go with single-minded, unnuanced applications of, say, utilitarian or deontological theory, running roughshod over that complexity and usually devoid of moral imagination and sensitivity.[12]

Even if it were possible to produce an ethical theory satisfying the criteria suggested by Callahan and discussed by Childress and Beauchamp, how successful would its application be in practice? Carl Elliott asserts that if the task/aim of applied ethics is to apply normative moral theories to ethical problems, then it does not work. He notes that 'the practical difficulty with applying ethical theories is that ordinary people pay little attention to theories when they make their moral decisions. Moral decisions are, of course, influenced often by theories of one sort or another, but this influence is usually indirect rather than explicit'.[13]

Our own experience of teaching medical ethics to doctors and nurses is that whilst one may present them with four principles as an ethical framework, and link the principles with the rules of established professional codes, health care professionals do not seem to 'use' the principles in the resolution of cases discussed immediately afterwards. Moreover, if one analyses a case simply in terms of principles, one is likely to overlook many details which are morally relevant. Simplifying a case so that it appears as a conflict between, for example, the principles of respect for autonomy and beneficence, may make it appear easier to resolve, but that appearance may be misleading and may hide morally important features of the case.

There are therefore difficulties in coming up with a satisfactory ethical theory, and in any case health care professionals are unlikely to use such a theory when resolving the moral problems of particular cases. The problem is really analogous to the one we have touched on earlier. The Hippocratic tradition seeks causal laws and interventions which can apply to all similar cases. Likewise, the Hippocratic ethical tradition seeks general theories, principles and rules, or most famously 'oaths' and 'codes', which can be universally applied. It is part of our critique that such general rules or principles cannot be applied in mechanical ways, and that there is no substitute for the individual doctor's or nurse's judgement in the particular ethical situation. This is not of course to say that these rules and principles are irrelevant, but rather that, in an Asklepian manner, their relevance to a particular case is what is important and requires judgement. The rules and principles cannot be used as premises from which, with some facts about individual cases, we can deduce the correct ethical answer. This position requires some development since the advocacy of this kind of approach to ethical decision-making is one aspect of our positive contribution to the reconstruction of palliative care.

The 'philosophy' of palliative care influences clinical practice—that is to say, it influences the decisions people actually make. If those decisions are made, as Elliott suggests, without explicit reference to ethical theory, then how are they made, and how does the expressed ideology of palliative care influence practice?

Whenever clinicians recognize a moral problem in a particular case, they describe the case to themselves, and, let us hope, to the rest of the team. This description is drawn against the background of the philosophy of palliative care which forms part of their cultural background and values. What part does the description of the case play in the resolution of the problem, and what part does the philosophy of palliative care play?

When faced with the task of sorting out what is wrong and what is to be done, health care practitioners first listen to the patient's story. The importance of listening to the patient's account has been much stressed recently in articles on 'narrative-based medicine'. This idea is not new, for the importance of 'taking a good history', which simply means listening carefully to the patient's own account, has been stressed in medical education for many years. Proponents of narrative-based medicine suggest that having listened attentively to that story, a professional interpretation of it is constructed and recorded.[14] The way that the story is described, interpreted, and recorded is part of the analysis of any moral problems inherent in the case.

Carl Elliott notes that 'the real work of bioethics, more often than not, is in listening, reading, and watching carefully in order to judge what is important and what is not'.[15] He goes on to stress that the way in which we recount the story of the case naturally plays into a certain way of thinking about it. He concludes that 'When we use language, we are not just representing the world; we are interpreting it, and in some ways, creating it.... the manner in which a bioethicist writes the case narrative—the setting, the narrator's voice, the use of irony and so on—will reflect his or her own philosophical arguments'.[16]

A purely objective presentation of a case is not possible, for such a presentation always entails inclusion of factors considered relevant and exclusion of others, plus some interpretation of the scenario presented. The language chosen greatly influences the way actions are interpreted: for example, in the context of palliative care removal of a life-prolonging treatment may variously be described as an act which allows the patient to die or an act which brings about the patient's death. The words used clearly indicate the author's own perspective. Elliott notes that what is problematic is not that narrative style communicates a personal moral vision, for this is obvious, but rather that the case presentation 'packages a personal moral vision in the surface wrapping of objectivity'.[17]

The way in which a case is described causes it to fall into a certain class of similar cases. This resembles the process of diagnosis itself; doctors make diagnoses by comparing the package of symptoms and signs with those typical of certain diseases, and deciding which disease the presenting package most resembles. They then conclude that the presenting illness is most likely to be a case of that disease, and treat it accordingly. When confronted with a moral problem in a case they will tend to react in the same way; they will gather together the features of the case they consider relevant, and then they will try to classify the case by deciding what general type of case it most resembles. How they classify the case will much depend on the words used in the description: for example, it may be seen as a case of either killing or letting die, or of a patient refusing a life-prolonging treatment or of a patient committing suicide. For each class of cases there will be a paradigm case, that is, a case which contains all the most important features, and one on which there is general agreement about the right course of action, rather in the same way as there is general agreement about the best treatment for a certain disease. When the problem case has been identified as similar in important ways to the paradigm case, doctors will tend to conclude that they should act in the way accepted as right for the paradigm case, unless of course there are certain features of the problem case which suggest otherwise.

This approach to moral problems has a long history. It developed in the early modern period and acquired the name of 'casuistry', a name which refers to the central role of paradigm cases in moral reasoning. It acquired a bad reputation, was heavily criticized and abandoned as a model of moral reasoning until recently. We should note here that it appeals to doctors as a method of moral reasoning because of its similarity to the process of diagnosis. This similarity was pointed out by Albert Jonsen and Stephen Toulmin in their book *The abuse of casuistry.*[18]

It is certainly true that doctors and nurses working in palliative care tend to identify a particular case with a paradigm case. For example, they might see the question of whether or not artificial hydration should be given to a dying patient as resembling a paradigm case of providing a treatment which will simply prolong dying. In contrast, their colleagues outside palliative care would be more likely to consider the case as resembling a paradigm where adequate hydration is considered essential to prolong or sustain life, as in acute care. So the way that doctors and nurses describe a particular case determines how they think it should be managed, for they tend to decide how to manage individual cases by considering how a similar but paradigm case would be managed. The philosophy of palliative care influences how professionals describe the ethical problems they recognize in individual cases.

This is an important point because it means that the moral reasoning of casuistry is not a value-neutral process. For instance, when professionals outside palliative care describe cases they tend to present the 'facts' of the case, but may omit details relating to the emotional impact of the situation on the patient, family and professionals. This omission occurs because such emotional issues are considered either as irrelevant, or even dangerous because they may cloud judgement; they are not part of the Hippocratic approach. In contrast, professionals working in palliative care are charged with maximising the patient's and family's psychological, spiritual and social well-being, and so they tend to include in their package of relevant features the emotional impact of the situation on all concerned. Such considerations are part of the Asklepian approach. In this way the philosophy of palliative care can influence professional decision-making.

It is debatable whether emotional engagement in the case story by professionals is dangerous or provides essential enlightenment. As Elliott notes, emotional engagement may either illuminate judgement or cloud it.[19] It is difficult to argue that moral judgement should be completely detached from sympathy and the imagination, but it is also clear that too much 'empathy' or 'suffering with' the patient may lead to personal emotional trauma and loss of ability to weigh up all the relevant features of the case. This latter possibility is discounted by some writers. Ann Scott considers it important to identify imaginatively with the patient, a process which she thinks will enable the doctor or nurse to understand what a particular treatment would be like for the patient.[20] This sort of approach is often encouraged in palliative care, but it is associated with risks of emotional distress sufficient to cloud the judgement of professionals (and also sufficient to lead to emotional exhaustion). We shall discuss this in more detail in Chapter 7. In the present context the important point is that the presentation of a case is not simply a matter of neutrally describing objective facts; it involves interpretation and therefore value judgements.

Moreover, the way a case is described and interpreted by professionals actually leads to their resolution of it, just as the description of symptoms and signs leads to diagnosis and treatment. When specialists in palliative care describe a case they will be influenced by their culture and values, and that culture and those values are currently strongly determined by the 'philosophy' described in the WHO statement. So the WHO philosophy of palliative care determines how specialists in the field perceive the moral issues which arise in palliative care. Such strongly held beliefs easily become pervasive.

Since these beliefs are not shared outside palliative care, specialists in palliative care frequently 'see' cases differently from their non-specialist colleagues, and hence often come to different conclusions about what is the right course of action. Thus patients in the care of specialists, for example in hospices, may well receive different treatment and care from those in the non-specialist setting. Specialists have tended to want to influence their colleagues in other settings to share their own beliefs and thus follow the pattern of their clinical practice, but would this be desirable? Health care aims to provide for each individual patient the best treatment and care in the particular circumstances. The WHO philosophy of palliative care, and the impact it has on clinical decisions, should be examined in order to determine whether its adoption more widely in health care would lead to better treatment of terminally ill patients.

1.9 Paradoxes in palliative care

It has been our contention in this chapter that the Hippocratic tradition of scientific medicine, including its ethical analogue of 'principlism', has joined forces with consumerism and together they have successfully colonized palliative medicine. This is illustrated in a number of paradoxes which we shall outline as a way of summing up the problems we intend to address in the body of our book.

Firstly, as we have seen, palliative care originated in very patient-centred values and ideas, and the origin of modern palliative care in Dame Cicely's vision was very Asklepian.[21] On the other hand, the specialty of palliative care has become increasingly Hippocratic. While there is an emphasis in the theory of palliative care on listening and communication skills, on concentrating attention on this individual patient, in practice structured interviews and questionnaires are advocated. This reality is summed up by that favourite term 'assessment tool'. The term expresses the sad delusion that, like the surgeon's scalpel, the assessment tool is in itself an effective intervention. In other words, palliative care professionals, instead of listening to the sick patient's needs, fears, and wishes, and accepting these at face value, are encouraged or exhorted to impose professional templates.

Secondly, whereas there is emphasis on patient autonomy and empower-ment, there is considerable paternalism. For example, there is stress on the necessity for psychosocial and spiritual assessment followed by interventions, whether the patient is seeking these or not. If patients do not seem to want these then they are 'holding back' or are 'in denial'.

Thirdly, as we noted above, there is great emphasis on 'patient-centredness' and patient choice. Nevertheless, the views and needs of relatives are given equal and sometimes even greater importance than those of patients in palliative care. The patient's wish to die at home, even in a house which they may wholly or partly own, may be denied at the request of relatives. Similarly the process of dying may be prolonged at the request of relatives and against the best interests of patients, and despite the doctrine we mention below that palliative care professionals neither hasten nor postpone death.

Fourthly, specialist palliative care has developed on the basis that there is a set of specialist knowledge and skills. But there is a parallel idea that this knowledge and these skills can be imparted to non-specialists - that every branch of health care can be taught appropriate end-of-life treatment which can achieve similar results. The WHO document, *Better palliative care for older people,* recommends that the care currently provided for cancer patients in hospices, 'now needs to be provided for those with a wider range of diseases'.[22] In other words, generalists, or specialists in other branches of health care, can and ought to follow the same philosophy and practice as has been developed in specialist palliative care. To what extent then, if at all, ought palliative care to be a specialty? We discuss this in Chapter 9.

Fifthly, the WHO further states: 'The idea that palliative care support and care should be offered alongside potentially curative treatment, although obvious to patients and families, appears a radical idea for some health professionals'.[23] It is certainly a radical idea to us, as it is logically impossible to provide simultaneously 'palliative' and 'curative' care.

Sixthly, whilst seeing itself as a branch of health care, palliative care simul-taneously distances itself from the ethos of health care by adopting different practices. For example, in the WHO definition (which we will discuss later) we are told that palliative care 'intends neither to hasten nor to prolong death'. Given that death occurs in a moment, this phrase must mean 'intends neither to hasten nor to prolong dying'. But conventional health care seeks to prolong life, until the moment of death. In conventional care dying patients would be offered certain life-prolonging treatments, such as intravenous hydration in irreversible intestinal obstruction. In contrast this would probably not be offered in specialist palliative care, as it would be seen as prolonging dying.

Moreover, in conventional health care psychosocial and spiritual care is not primarily undertaken by health care professionals—and indeed is not seen as part of health care at all. But palliative care emphasizes that psychosocial and spiritual care are part of the remit of health care professionals, possibly because they are thought to contribute to quality of life, and to one ideal of a 'good death'. Here again, palliative care is different from conventional health care.

Finally, despite the emphasis on patient autonomy or choice, palliative care professionals (in the UK at least) are opposed to euthanasia and physician-assisted suicide even if patients favour these procedures. We are not, by any means, advocating these practices but simply pointing out that in a philosophy which so heavily stresses patient-centredness and patient self-determination and choice it is hardly consistent to react so strongly against those who advocate euthanasia or physician-assisted suicide.

These are just some of the paradoxes and problems we have found in the philosophy and practice of palliative care. They will be discussed in more detail in various contexts, although not in any particular order.

We must repeat here that we believe that the palliative care movement is profoundly important for modern health care. Our intention is to strip away the rhetoric found in the philosophy statements and in some of the research. The root of the problem may be that those in palliative care are trying too hard and have become over-professionalized. A symptom of this is the extraordinary claim made in the current WHO definition of palliative care. The definition tells us that those in palliative care can offer an 'impeccable' assessment and treatment of pain and other symptoms. This is embarrassing rhetoric! The reality is that the dedicated members of palliative teams do their very best to offer a high standard of care to very sick patients, but which of us can say that our assessments and treatments are 'impeccable'? Certainly it is important that the Hippocratic techniques of modern medicine should be available in palliative care as in other areas of health care. But the Asklepian moment, the concentrated attention, the quietness, flow more authentically from the professional's own humanity than from externally imposed guidelines, protocols, scales, and assessments.

1.10 **Conclusions**

1 The practice of palliative care as it was developed by Dame Cicely Saunders in St Christopher's in the 1960s had its origins in a medieval tradition of

care for the dying and an even older Greek medical tradition which we have associated with the shadowy figure of Asklepius. This practice has been condensed into the WHO 'definition' of palliative care.

2 The early traditions of palliative care have been re-interpreted in terms of the interventionist approaches of scientific medicine, initiated by Hippocrates, with its stress on generalizability and measurable outcomes.

3 The result has been a distortion of the original Asklepian approach as developed in the modern world by Dame Cicely Saunders. This distortion has resulted in a number of paradoxes.

4 The distortion extends even to the area of ethics where the wrong kind of emphasis on generalizations, rules, and principles has blinded practitioners to the importance of the individual case.

5 As a positive contribution we have suggested a case-based approach to ethical decision-making, an approach which is congruent with the way in which health professionals approach diagnosis and treatment.

References

1 Roy, D. J. (2004). Humanity: image, idea, reality. *Journal of Palliative Care*, 20(3): 131–2.
2 Macklin, R. (2003). Dignity is a useless concept. *BMJ*, 327: 1419–20.
3 WHO (2002). *National cancer control programes: policies and managerial guidelines*, 2nd edn. WHO, Geneva.
4 Saunders, C. (2003). *Watch with me*. Mortal Press, Sheffield: p. 46.
5 Southgate, M. T. (1997). *The art of JAMA*. Mosby, St Louis, MO: p. xii.
6 Kaasa, S. and Loge, J.H. (2004). Quality of life in palliative medicine/principles and practice. In: *Oxford textbook of palliative medicine*, 3rd edn, ed. D. Doyle, G. Hanks, N. Cherny, *et al*. Oxford University Press, Oxford: pp. 196–210.
7 World Health Organization (1946). *Constitution*. WHO, New York.
8 Elliott, C. (1999). *A philosophical disease*. Routledge, New York: p. xix.
9 Elliott, C. (1999). op. cit. p. xxxi.
10 Elliott, C. (1999). op. cit. p. xxxiv.
11 Childress, J. and Beauchamp, T. (1994). Types of Ethical Theory. In: *Principles of biomedical ethics*, 4th edn. Oxford University Press, Oxford: pp. 100–111.
12 Callahan, D. (2000). *Universalism and particularism: fighting to a draw*. Hastings Centre Report 30, no. 1: 37–44.
13 Elliott, C. (1999). op. cit. p. 148.
14 Greenhalgh, T. (1998). Narrative based medicine in an evidence based world. In: *Narrative based medicine*, ed. T. Greenhalgh and B. Hurwitz. BMJ Books, London: p. 258.
15 Elliott, C. (1999). op. cit. p. xxvi.
16 Elliott, C. (1999). op. cit. p. 123.
17 Elliott, C. (1999). op. cit. p. 125.
18 Jonsen, A. and Toulmin, S. (1998). *The abuse of casuistry*. California University Press, Los Angeles, CA: pp. 36–46.

19 Elliott, C. (1999). op. cit. p. 127.
20 Scott, A. (1998). Nursing, narrative and the moral imagination. In: *Narrative based medicine* op. cit., p. 152.
21 Clark, D. (2002). Between hope and acceptance: the medicalisation of dying. *BMJ*, **324**: 905–7.
22 WHO (2004). *Better palliative care for older people.* WHO, Geneva: p. 8.
23 WHO (2004). op. cit. p. 17.

2

Quality of life

Introduction

The concept of quality of life is central to the philosophy of palliative care. Indeed, it is given pride of place in the WHO definition of palliative care. The authors of the chapter on quality of life in the *OTPM* go one step further, maintaining that quality of life was the goal of medicine in the Greek world (and they cite Aristotle in support) and has been the goal of medicine ever since.[1] This suggestion is completely incorrect. To the extent that the Greeks had a single view of the goal of medicine—and as we have seen there was both an Asklepian and a Hippocratic tradition—it is stated by Hippocrates thus: 'the complete removal of the distress of the sick, the alleviation of the more violent diseases and the refusal to undertake to cure cases in which the disease has already won the mastery, knowing that everything is not possible to medicine'.[2]

This realistic aim does not even hint at quality of life! Moreover, the passage cited from Aristotle in the *OTPM* has nothing whatsoever to do with medicine—it is concerned with the aim of political science. More tellingly, the authors note that between 1961and 1965 there were no entries indexed at all in Medline under the keyword 'quality of life', whereas between 1996 and 2000 there were 12, 749.[3] In other words, the idea that 'quality of life' is the 'overall goal' in health care, or more modestly, is a helpful concept, is entirely a product of medical and nursing thinking in the second half of the twentieth century. Our central aim in this chapter is to discuss the extent to which it has been a helpful concept, especially in palliative care.

Of course, it might be said that while Hippocrates states the aims of medicine in a specific way, the ultimate point of pursuing these specific aims is to improve quality of life. In a similar way, the orthopaedic surgeon might say that his aim in carrying out a hip replacement is to improve quality of life. Yes, but the trouble with this move is that it is too successful! It can be said of any occupational activity whatsoever! Thus, the aim of the gardener is to grow good flowers and vegetables and so improve our quality of life; the aim of the policeman is to protect us from criminals, and so improve our quality of life. In other words, to claim that some occupational activity is to improve quality of life is entirely unhelpful unless we are also told how specifically this is going to be done.

It follows that if health care professionals, patients, their families and the community are to have some shared understanding of the philosophy and aims of palliative care, then a clear, shared and specific concept of 'quality of life' is essential. The first question is whether such a clear and shared concept exists now or could be developed.

The achievement of explicit goals is the measure of success of a health care service or treatment. When decisions are made regarding either the funding of services and treatments or the appropriateness of treatments for individual patients, the evidence regarding the success of those services and treatments must be considered. If the success of palliative care services or palliative treatments in achieving their explicit goal is to be assessed, then it must be possible to assess whether quality of life has been improved for the patient and family. The second question is whether it is possible to assess quality of life, either by measurement or by the provision of qualitative information on specific treatments.

It is often claimed that quality of life studies can improve decision making for individual patients. Our third question is whether that is in fact the case. If, following discussion, the thesis is accepted that quality of life as a global concept should not be used, then a fourth question is posed - what should be the aim(s) or goal(s) of palliative care?

Even if we assume that palliative care can improve quality of life, we must still face a final question: can palliative care improve quality of life more than conventional services and alternative models of treatment, and if so, is it cost effective? Since discussion of this issue requires consideration of the principles of resource allocation it will be discussed in Chapter 8. We have, then, four questions in this chapter and they will be discussed in order.

- Is there a clear and shared concept of quality of life, and if not, could one be developed?
- Can quality of life be assessed by measurement, or is it preferable to use domain-specific qualitative studies?
- Do quality of life assessments improve decision making for individual patients?
- If 'quality of life' is rejected as the aim of palliative care what should its aim be?

2.1 The use of the term 'quality of life'

Awareness of mortality is heightened in the context of a terminal illness, and it is perhaps this inescapable and inevitable link between the fact of mortality and ideas of 'living well' that contributes to the importance placed on quality of life for patients and their families in palliative care. When it is clear that little life remains, and loss of present opportunity cannot be compensated by future actions, patients and all around them become focused on achieving the ideal of the best possible quality for the remaining life. But, more specifically, what is meant by improving quality of life?

The term 'quality of life' has become part of the English language, and is now commonly used both within health care and also in daily life. Many writers note the fact that no satisfactory definition of quality of life has been produced, but judging by the volume of literature on the topic, the search for one has not been abandoned. Yet it is possible to explain why a helpful definition cannot be found, even in principle. Since this is highly relevant to our argument in this chapter we shall try to untangle some of the complexities in the term which make it impossible to define, even in principle.

2.1.1 Qualities, evaluations, and definability

Firstly, a 'quality' can mean simply an attribute, a characteristic, or a disposition of something or someone. In this sense the term 'quality' is purely descriptive of some fact or identifiable state of affairs, and is therefore evaluatively neutral. For example, cooking apples will have certain qualities or characteristics, such as being of a certain size, cooking well, and having a sharp flavour. Again, types of disease will be associated with certain characteristics, symptoms, or qualities, such as breathlessness or nausea, while a psychopath will be disposed to act in certain ways or will have certain qualities. The first requirement of a quality of life judgement, then, is that it must be grounded in descriptively-identifiable factual qualities.

This may seem too obvious to state, but, as we shall see, there are those who wish to base quality of life judgements simply on how the patient claims to feel. How the patient feels is certainly an important consideration, but it is not the only factor relevant to a quality of life judgement. To the extent that a quality is present, some factual, or objectively identifiable, factor must be present. In the context of quality of life judgements in health care typical qualities which are factually identifiable might be nausea, breathlessness, mobility, capacity to respond to questions, and so on.

Secondly, when we use the term 'quality of life', as distinct from the term 'quality' on its own, we are making a judgement which evaluates these factual qualities. In other words, we are standing back from the factual qualities we have noted and assessing them as good or poor. The quality of life judgement is an assessment which is consequential on, or results from, the identification of the list of relevant factual qualities. To put this another way, we might say that 'quality of life' is not another item on a list which includes factual qualities such as nausea or mobility; rather it is a value judgement resulting from a total assessment of the qualities on the list.

The point that quality of life judgements are value judgements about factual qualities and not in themselves factual qualities is not always appreciated. We have found that some researchers use the term 'quality of life' as if it itself were a factual quality or set of qualities. For example, in a study 'to determine the association between symptoms and depression in patients with advanced cancer' Professor Mari Lloyd-Williams et al. include a table detailing the following items, each of which receives a score: pain, mood, breathlessness, physical movement, general quality of life, and tiredness. The point the authors have missed is that 'general quality of life' is not an item like the others. The others are descriptive or factual qualities, and 'general quality of life' ought not to be a separate item on that list; rather it is consequential on the others.[4]

A similar error is to be found in a discussion of 'dignity and psychothera-peutic considerations in end-of life care'. Dr Harvey Max Chochinov et al. state that 'A factor analysis of the dignity data set yielded six primary factors, including: 1) pain; 2) intimate dependency; 3) hopelessness/depression; 4) informal support network; 5) formal support network; and 6) quality of life.[5]

The point however is that items 1–5 are factual, descriptive, objective factors, whereas the all-things-considered quality of life judgement results from a survey of these facts (by the patient or professional) and is an evaluation of the quality of life as good or poor, granted the five (or more) factors to be found in the life.

The mistake of placing quality of life on the same list as the objective factors such as pain, depression, support etc. amounts to what philosophers call a 'category mistake'.[6] To illustrate, let us suppose a visitor to the University of Oxford visits the Colleges and at the end of the day says, 'I've seen the Colleges, but where is the University?'. That is a category mistake, for the University is the sum total of the Colleges. In a similar way, 'quality of life' judgements (logically) must be assessments resulting from the sum total of the factors surveyed.

To summarize so far, we are saying that there are two elements in quality of life judgements: there must be identifiable, factual qualities; and there must be an evaluation of these identifiable factors as comprising a good or poor quality of life.

There are however other complications which arise in the making of quality of life judgements. Firstly, the list of qualities, in the descriptive, identifiable sense, that people might value in their lives is obviously very large, and we can never be sure we have noted them all on our list. For example, people might value having friends, being at home, being able to listen to music, having a job, and so on. The number of possible items which could be included on this list is enormous. Secondly, the emphases (or evaluations) which different people might place on different items will vary. Moreover, even the same people might place a different value on different factors at different times in their lives.

It should now be clear why 'quality of life' cannot be defined in any strict sense of definition. Firstly, since the list of identifiable qualities relevant to a quality of life assessment for a given person is very large we can never be sure we have listed them all. Secondly, the items which different people might consider relevant to an assessment will vary. Thirdly, even the same person may stress different factors as relevant over a period of a month. Quality of life cannot therefore be defined, not because it is difficult to do but because it is logically impossible. Attempts to define it should simply be abandoned.

We recognize that this conclusion is controversial. In the *OTPM*, Stein Kaasa and Jon Havard Loge argue that health-related quality of life is an abstract concept, and that 'in order to communicate about an abstract phenomenon, one needs to agree upon a definition of the concept, how to explore the concept, and how to summarize the findings. In other words, an accurate description of a subjective phenomenon depends upon how the concept is defined, how data is collected, processed, and communicated'.[7] Our position is that definition of the concept is not possible. This leads to the conclusion that data encompassing it cannot be collected, processed, or communicated.

2.1.2 The global sense of quality of life

Now it by no means follows, from anything we have said so far, that the WHO philosophy is mistaken in making its central aim the attainment for patients of an improved quality of life. For it might be said that, whereas the list of qualities which patients might value in their lives is very large, the qualities can mainly be placed under certain headings. In more detail, it would be possible to draw up a typical list of factors which many people would consider important for an overall good quality of life. For example, most people would mention being healthy, having a job, a decent income, having friends, living in a safe and pleasant environment, having some leisure, being able to make a few choices about one's life, and so on. There is absolutely no difficulty in compiling such a list and finding wide agreement about the items which should be on it. Difficulty arises only if we claim that we have an exhaustive list—for it is easy to omit an item which is crucial to the quality of life of a given person—or if we try to rank the items in any order of importance—for different people stress different items on the list, and a given person's view of the items may change with time and circumstances. Hence, while it is not possible even in principle to produce an agreed overall definition of quality of life in this broad sense, we can formulate lists of typical factors which we all might like to have in our lives. In this way the term 'quality of life' might still be a helpful one in health assessments.

This is the line taken by Lesley Fallowfield, a lecturer in psychology also qualified as a nurse and counsellor, in her book *The quality of life: the missing measurement in health care*.[8] Fallowfield's purpose is to stress the importance of looking at the overall effects of treatment on the patient, especially in those circumstances where the benefit of prolonging life may be outweighed by the unpleasant aspects of treatment and continued existence in a state of disease or disability with no prospect of restoration to health. Her book is not written with the aim of influencing resource allocation, but in order to make health care professionals and the public more aware of the overall effects of treatment so that better individual treatment decisions might be made. Her work is particularly relevant to palliative care, not least because her inspiration for studying the subject was her observations of the adverse effects of palliative chemotherapy on a close friend, which stimulated her to look particularly at quality at the end of life.

Since she considers explicit definition to be a pre-requisite for measurement, she is committed to producing a definition, which is the following: quality of life is a 'complex amalgam of satisfactory functioning in essentially four core or primary domains' which are then listed as psychological, social, occupational, and physical.[9]

We might try to sum up Fallowfield's position by saying that she is using 'quality of life' in a broad or global sense; that she thinks that the many qualities people value in their lives can be placed under certain headings; that in this way the term can be defined (and measured); and that for these reasons it is a useful or central one in health care.

We have already discussed the issue of the indefinable nature of 'quality of life' so will not press the point again against Fallowfield (and we shall take up the point about measurement later). Let us rather consider the more important point of whether quality of life in her broad or global sense can be the central aim of palliative care, as the WHO philosophy suggests. Here it is relevant to make two points. Firstly, whatever health care is provided, the patient's (and family's) overall or global quality of life is outside the control of the health care team, and so the team cannot take responsibility for it. Our justification for this claim is that many of the factors of quality of life in the broader sense, such as satisfaction in employment or relationships, are not determined by health, which is neither necessary nor sufficient for their achievement. These factors are outside the remit of health care.

The second point in our reponse is that those providing and funding health care should recognize the responsibility of patients and their families for their own global quality of life, and should respect their privacy in governing their own lives. Thus those involved in health care should not endeavour to interfere in those factors related to overall quality of life which are not directly determined by or strongly influenced by health. Hence, it is often argued, as in the *OTPM*, that health care professionals should concentrate on health-related quality of life. In the relevant discussion on 'Quality of life in palliative medicine—principles and practice' the focus throughout is on 'Health-related quality of life—HRQOL'. Stein Kaasa and Jon Havard Loge note that:

> By reviewing the definition of the concept [HRQOL] it is clear that the content is highly influenced by setting, that is, the severity of physical symptoms, general health, spirituality, coping, existentially etc. However, there is general agreement to include at least symptomatology, physical, psychological, and social domains into the measures, although in many circumstances existential and spiritual domains also seem appropriate to include.'[10]

Whilst they note the agreement to include psychological and social domains, the emphasis throughout the extensive discussion is on methods to assess aspects of life seen to directly influence health, and their search is for an instrument to measure HRQOL during end of life care. They make no pretence to seek to measure the patient's overall quality of life.

2.1.3 Health-related quality of life

The idea of health-related quality of life arose historically when unpleasant life-prolonging treatments first became available for illnesses such as cancer—one often heard patients and health care professionals say that in the context of a terminal illness it is 'quality of life that matters, not quantity'. Similarly, some authors have noted that the most appropriate aim for health care is 'not to add years to life, but life to years'.[11] Such statements arose from the realization that prolonging a life characterized by pain and other symptoms, plus perhaps disability and dependency, without hope of restoration of health, might not constitute an overall benefit to the patient.

In her book, *Measuring health: a review of quality of life measurement scales*, Ann Bowling, a medical sociologist, acknowledges that the conceptualization and measurement of the outcomes or consequences of health care are controversial.

However, she states that 'There is now a recognition that meaningful measures of *health-related quality of life* [our italics] should be used to evaluate health care interventions', and that 'In order to measure health outcome a measure of health status is required which in turn must be based on a concept of health'.[12]

Bowling notes that health status should take into account two concepts: firstly, that of 'disease' which is a pathological abnormality indicated by a set of signs and symptoms, and secondly, the person's 'ill health' which is indicated by feelings such as pain or perceptions of change in usual functioning and feeling. A general statement about the importance of the patient's subjective experience follows:

> What matters in the 20th century is how the patient feels, rather than how doctors think they ought to feel on the basis of clinical measurements. Symptom response or survival rates are no longer enough; and, particularly where people are treated for chronic or life-threatening conditions, the therapy has to be evaluated in terms of whether it is more or less likely to lead to an outcome of a life worth living in social and psychological, as well as physical, terms.[13]

There is a current fashion in health care and health care ethics for considering that the only factor of importance in health status or in the outcome of health care is how the patient feels, and that other evidence, even that which is uncontroversial such as whether the patient is alive or dead, is simply irrelevant. This makes little sense. Moreover, the term 'feels' is ambiguous and might refer to bodily sensations of discomfort or to unhappiness at one's lot in life. Bowling's initial implication that what matters is only how the patient feels must be rejected.

We have already made it clear in Section 2.1.1 that if the term 'quality of life' is to be used then objective qualities must be present—it is not just a matter of the patient's subjective feelings. Indeed, if the patient's subjective feelings are to be the only or the main determinants of the care offered then we could simply drop entirely the term 'quality of life' and just ask patients how they feel about a treatment. There is a case for taking this line, but what cannot consistently be done is to hold on to the term 'quality of life' and also to maintain that the only or the main factor in determining this is how the patient feels.

Ann Bowling claims that there are essentially two parts to the concept of health-related quality of life. The first includes functional ability, which is to do with being able to carry out the acts of self-care and domestic activity, as well as functional status which is directly related to the ability to perform social roles. The second part is a concept of positive health, which implies 'full-functioning' or 'efficiency' of mind, body, and social adjustment, as well as the related concepts of social well-being and quality of life which she sees as components of a broad concept of positive health.[14]

One must conclude from her description of these two parts of the concept of health-related quality of life that it is a very broad theory indeed. It includes many characteristics of life which are not solely or principally determined by health, as well as concepts for which there are no generally accepted comprehensive definitions or descriptions. This apparently unsatisfactory conclusion is inevitable, for there simply is no comprehensive and coherent description of the concept of health-related quality of life, with clear boundaries between it and non-health-related quality of life.

> Another attempt to limit quality of life judgements to 'health related quality of life' is to be found in the *OTPM*. The authors of the relevant chapter write that 'Despite the ongoing discussion about how to define QOL, most researchers and clinicians agree that QOL in palliative medicine is related to symptom control, physical function, psychological well being, and meaning and fulfilment (existential and spiritual issues). This multidimentional health-oriented concept has been named by many clinicians and researchers as health-related quality of life, HRQOL'.[15]

The trouble with this list is that, while there are not many items on it, it is anything but narrow! No one could possibly quarrel with the idea that symptom control, physical function, and perhaps, depending on what we are going to mean by the term, psychological well-being, are central to a patient's quality of life in palliative care, and are on the whole manageable objectives for the professionals involved. But what are we to make of 'meaning and fulfilment (existential and spiritual issues)'? In the first place, meaning and fulfilment are enormously broad issues—nothing could be more global—since they involve a whole lifetime, and issues well outside health care. Secondly, such matters cannot be dealt with satisfactorily in the few weeks a patient may be receiving palliative care, and it may simply make matters worse to take the lid off problems which may have been simmering for years. Of course, if a patient wishes to discuss matters with a clergyman then this is entirely appropriate, but it is not a matter for health care professionals. This is a controversial position to adopt, and we shall discuss it further in Chapter 7. But to those outside palliative care it seems astonishing, and incredibly paternalistic, that professionals whose qualifications are in nursing or social work should feel confident enough to make the meaning of and fulfilment in the patient's life an aim of their health care.

Of course, it might be argued that a distinction should be drawn between dealing with meaning and fulfiment as such, and dealing with them to the extent that they impact on quality of life or general well being. In other words, the objection is that even health-related quality of life is determined by factors other than physical illness, or that factors in the broader concept of global quality of life are bound to affect those in the narrower one of health-related quality of life. Meaning and fulfilment might then be said to be factors relevant to palliative care since they may affect psychological well being and possibly also the 'total pain' spoken about by Dame Cicely Saunders.[16]

In reply to this we shall make two points. Firstly, many professionals in palliative care are concerned with meaning and fulfilment for their own sake. What lies behind this is some general philosophical or religious position about a 'good death'. It is as if the religious roots of palliative care in religious houses and hospices—where the confession of sins and absolution were requisites of a good death—have been grafted on to a secular philosophy to the effect that an 'authentic' death requires that one puts everything right. Our reply to this is simply that not everyone wishes this kind of end, and those who do are likely to be much better served by the clergy than palliative care professionals.

Secondly, even if these profound matters do affect health it seems to show grotesque disrespect to their importance to deal with them for the sake of a patient's health-related quality of life. Is a person's awe or fear at the prospect of entering the presence of God to be allayed by someone who has done a course in counselling? Or who has read a book on fulfilment in life? Or who knows what 'existential' means? In sum, the most important point is that it is belittling the universally acknowledged importance to human beings of the meaning of life to see it as one factor in 'health-related quality of life'. It is even more ludicrous to attempt to put a score on this. Readers should be reminded of Douglas Adams' 1979 novel, *The hitchhiker's guide to the galaxy*, where the meaning of life is given as 42. We all accept that this is ludicrous and therefore funny, but quality of life, or spirituality, as a single scored item is equally ludicrous. And yet there are attempts to devise such scales.[17]

As we have indicated, this position is controversial, and further discussion arises in Chapter 4 in relation to care of the relatives, and in Chapter 7 in relation to psychosocial care. And while we have not raised the matter of resources in this chapter we shall argue that any health service, whether funded by taxation, voluntary contributions, or insurance policies, must use its resources fairly (see Chapter 8). It is not at all clear that grandiose aims, such as dealing with meaning and fulfilment in people's lives, should be funded from health care resources.

Our first question in this chapter was whether there exists a shared conception of quality of life, or if one could be developed. Our answer is that there is not a shared conception, either in ordinary or in professional discourse. The attempt to develop one via the apparently more limited idea of 'health-related quality of life' also fails. The list of items on it is much more restricted, but some, such as meaning in life and fulfilment, lie well outside the scope of health care. We now turn to the second issue—the success or failure of the many attempts to assess and measure the poorly identified concept of quality of life.

2.2 Assessment and measurement of quality of life

There is a prevailing view in health care that however difficult the project we simply must provide measurement of the impact of health care on quality of life. There are three good thoughts behind the measurement imperative. Firstly, it is considered that if scarce resources are to be expended to best effect and distributed justly, then we need to be able to compare the outcome of one service or treatment with another. Secondly, it may be argued that measurement/assessment of quality of life might enable better care to be provided for individual patients, for example by using the assessment tool to identify the patient's subjective symptoms.[18] Thirdly, there is a current enthusiasm for expressing everything as a number or statistic, which is associated with a lack of regard for the results of qualitative research not presented numerically. The consequence of these strong trends is an overwhelming drive to establish quality of life measurement techniques and scales. The use of such a scale in every clinical trial of a service or treatment is now considered essential. The chapter on quality of life in the *OTPM* carries discussion of many measurement scales and the criteria they must satisfy.

It is interesting that this drive has persisted despite obvious problems in measuring quality of life in terms of the theory of measurement. These problems are grave, and appear insurmountable. It is surprising that despite acknowledgement of this difficulty sociologists, statisticians, and health care professionals persist in the belief that it is possible to overcome them, and they continue to try to measure quality of life.

2.2.1 Theory of measurement and quality of life

Measurement tools must meet certain criteria in order to be considered acceptable for research purposes. These criteria include validity and reliability, and tests to demonstrate validity and reliability have been established. These are set out and discussed in the *OTPM* and many other places. Conclusions drawn from invalid measurement tools are themselves invalid, therefore measurement tools failing to meet these criteria should be rejected. But there is a more fundamental question underlying that of the validity of measurement tools: what is measurement, and can quality of life be measured even in principle?

Measurement is the act of attaching a number to an entity which is not itself a number. In using tools which measure quality of life a number is used to represent the patient's quality of life. We use numbers in three distinct ways, as described by Downie and Macnaughton in their book on clinical judgement.[19]

The first is as a method of identification or labelling. For example, after a clinical trial the state of the patient could be identified as either alive or dead and a number, such as 1 or 2 could be used to identify that state. The number in this case is simply serving as a sort of short-hand label, and this is not really a measurement as that concept is commonly understood. However, Bowling calls this a 'nominal' or 'classification' scale and describes it as the weakest form of measurement.[20] She asserts that there are methods of data transformation which permit even this use of numbers as labels, 'nominal data', to be made quantitative for the purposes of analysis. Yet as Downie and Macnaughton point out, the numbers used as labels have no relationship with each other and they are assigned in a totally arbitrary fashion. For instance, 'dead' could be 1 and 'alive' 2, or any other numbers we choose. It is simply not plausible to assert that numbers used simply as labels can be made into quantitative data, since the numbers put into the initial calculations do not represent a quantity—they are serving only as identifying symbols. It is not reasonable to suggest that from numbers used as labels any quantitative data can ever be obtained. Indeed, letters (A or B) could equally be used as labels.

The second use of numbers is to indicate the position of something in a series. Bowling calls this an 'ordinal' or ranking scale, and points out that many health-status measures are strictly of this type. The Karnofsky Performance scale rates physical ability between 0 and 100.[21] On this scale: 0 indicates that the patient is dead; a disabled patient requiring special care and assistance is 40; a patient's normal activity with effort is 80; and 100 is a normal patient with no complaints. These numbers are simply placing the patients' abilities in order; rating a patient's ability at 40 does not mean that the ability rated 40 is half as good as that rated at 80, or that being normal is one hundred times as good as being dead! The points on this scale are identified with numbers which happen to be separated by intervals of 10. This gives the impression that one state is ten units of something better than the state below, and that the difference between each state and its neighbours is the same. This is misleading, as the numbers are simply ranking disability (or ability).

Downie and Macnaughton point out that:

> when qualities are arranged in a series and identified with numbers, the use of those numbers to perform calculations like averages or percentages is meaningless, as the relationship between points 1 and 2 and between 5 and 6 in the series may be completely different. Distinctions between qualitative entities can very often only be expressed through descriptions like 'more and less' or 'better and worse' as they have no true numerical meaning.[22]

Despite this convincing argument attempts have been made to convert descriptions of entities into numerical scores on ordinal scales which are then subjected to statistical analysis. For example, a patient might be asked, 'Do you feel depressed?' and the patient ticks one of four possible response categories, such as 'very much', 'moderately', 'somewhat', or 'not at all'. These responses are each given a score from 0 to 3 or 0 to 4. Offering too few response categories, for example just yes and no, produces too crude a scale and insufficient opportunity for the patient to express his opinion accurately. On the other hand offering too many categories makes it difficult for patients to discriminate between categories.[23]

When the measurement tool requires patients to answer a number of items grouped into subsets, and the scores for all the subsets are added together, this is called a Likert scale. It must be noted that such a scale is at best producing an ordinal or ranking result. The patients have not assigned any number to their response—this is done by the test scorer—they have instead chosen a statement which most agrees with their own view. It cannot be assumed that a score of 4 for 'very much' is twice as bad as a score of 2 representing 'somewhat', or that the distance between 0 and 1 equals that between 3 and 4. All one can really say is that the patient is indicating progressively more depression from the 'not at all response' to the 'very much' response.

A striking example of this problem is provided by the 'Demoralization Scale' devised by David W. Kissane *et al.* and described in an article in the *Journal of Palliative Care* in 2004.[24] Patients answered questions regarding the frequency of feelings such as 'My life seems to be pointless' and indicated that frequency as 'never, seldom, sometimes, often and all the time'. The researchers then allocated the numbers 0, 1, 2, 3, and 4 respectively to these descriptive terms relating to frequency and complex statistical analysis was carried out on the numerical 'results'. But it is surely not reasonable to assume that 'all the time' yielding a score of 4 is twice as bad as 'sometimes' yielding a score of 2! The same problem applies to Guttman scales in which patients make a 'yes' or 'no' response to various items grouped together in degrees of severity, and the responses are scored 0 to 3 or 0 to 4.

Bowling is aware of the problems of subjecting data from ordinal scales to statistical analysis. She notes that the most appropriate statistic to draw from ordinal scales is the median, where the number of scores above and below the median is the same and the median itself is not altered by what those scores actually are. She writes later that summing up scores from two or more ordinal scales 'erroneously converts what is at best ordinal data into interval levels of measurement when applying statistical techniques. Statistical caution is required'.[25] Unfortunately quality of life measures require the scoring of several sorts of entities (such as mood, symptoms, and self-esteem) on ordinal scales and then adding together the results and subjecting them to statistical analysis. This is clearly an invalid process and it is difficult to see how even 'statistical caution' could render the results valid.

The third use of numbers is to describe a quantitative relationship between entities, which Bowling calls an 'interval' scale. The items on the scale are arranged in a series, as on the ordinal scale, but in addition it is known that the distances between any two numbers on the scale are of a known size. Usually they are the same size—the exception would be logarithmic scales. On the interval scale there is a constant unit of measurement, and so we can assign a 'real number' to the entity being measured. It should be noted that zero may be arbitrary, for example the centigrade and Fahrenheit temperature scales have arbitrary zero points since on neither scale does zero represent the complete absence of heat. Downie and Macnaughton describe entities which can be measured in this way as 'additive'.[26] A 'ratio' scale is like an interval scale but there is a true zero point, such as in weight when zero is scored when there is, in theory, no mass at all. A measurement of blood sugar or the entities of a full blood count are ratio scales as it is possible (in theory) to have no white blood cells or no blood glucose. The interval scale is truly quantitative and can be used for entities whose scores can be added together. All the common statistics such as means and standard deviations are applicable.

The obvious problem for quality of life tools is that the entities being measured, such as physical performance, role performance, mood, and social support can be represented on an ordinal scale but cannot be represented on an interval scale, since it cannot be said that a constant unit of measurement separates each point on the scale. As Bowling says, 'The most rigorous methods of data analysis require quantitative data. Whenever possible, measures which yield interval or ratio data should be used, although this is often difficult in social science. Measures of functional disability and health status never strictly reach a ratio- or interval-scale of measurement'.[27]

However, she goes on to assert that methods of data transformation permit even nominal data (and by implication also ordinal data) to be made quantitative for the purposes of analysis. If an entity is such that it simply cannot be measured on an interval scale, but only on an ordinal scale, surely no method of 'data transformation' can enable one to obtain the valid statistical data that can be derived only from data which can be legitimately represented on an interval scale.

Information about the domains of life thought relevant to measurement of quality of life is inherently qualitative (as opposed to quantitative) in nature. This gives rise to two problems relating to the use of ordinal scales. The first is that it is open to question whether such information can even be represented on an ordinal scale. The second is that in trying to represent it only by a number the information is diluted, weakened, or impoverished in some way. These problems arise persistently when attempts are made to represent entities such as mood or acceptance of dying on an ordinal scale.

The first problem is well illustrated and acknowledged by John Hinton in his paper on the awareness and acceptance of dying. His research was conducted by interviewing patients and relatives and scoring their level of acceptance between 1 and 9 depending on the phrases they used to describe their thoughts. Acceptance ratings between 1 and 4 'represented degrees of troubled rejection of a fatal outcome', ratings of 5 were 'noncommittal', and ratings between 6 and 9 indicated 'increasingly positive acceptance'. Some examples of brief quotations, with their ratings, for the full interview are listed below:

Rated 2 'I'm frightened he won't get better' (said with agitation and tears).
Rated 3 'I feel depressed, lonely at night. I cry if I talk about it.'
Rated 5 'I want to stay hopeful and don't want to look much farther.'
Rated 7 'I'm rather resigned to the situation.'
Rated 8 'I've got no fear of death, I've had my life—what happens after that who knows?'
Rated 9 'We both know all about it, it's accepted as God's will.'[28]

It is clear that this data can be presented only on an ordinal scale, for it is not possible to assert that there is a standard unit of difference of acceptance between each state. Indeed, one might consider that such descriptions are not always amenable even to an ordinal scale, for it is surely a matter of opinion whether the statement rated 3 above actually shows more acceptance than that rated 2. Hinton acknowledges this difficulty, explaining that 'Certain phrases about ways of accepting death became familiar and fell into clusters which help describe the ways that people saw their situation. These clusters were not clearly demarcated one from another'. If the clusters are not clearly demarcated one must question whether the descriptive phrases can be represented on an ordinal scale at all. Perhaps, if one must use numbers, all one can legitimately achieve is to attach a number as a label to each cluster of phrases, yielding only a nominal scale.

Despite the ordinal nature of the data Hinton still subjected it to statistical analysis; he states that the mean weekly score for acceptance increased from 7.0 eight weeks before the patients' deaths to 7.5 in the week before death, and quotes a $P < 0.05$. In so doing he has definitely (and erroneously) converted what is at best ordinal data into interval data, (the problem identified by Bowling and mentioned above).

The second problem, that of trying to represent a statement said in a certain way and in a context by a single numerical score, is also appreciated by Hinton. In the same paper he says: 'During interviews, measuring acceptance by quantitative ratings alone could seem as incomplete as estimating illumination in candlepower. Most people indicated or explained the nature and quality of their acceptance'. The analogy with illumination is powerful, for who would consider that the quality of moonlight could be represented by the numerical value of its candlepower!

The attempt to reduce the meaning of the patients' phrases to a numerical score greatly impoverishes our understanding of what they were trying to communicate. Thus much can be lost in the drive to obtain quantitative results from studies of entities which can be adequately represented only in language. Hinton does realize this, for he writes:

> The shaping of questions and measurements to give standardised and more reliable answers is necessary for research, but it may limit or distort people's self-descriptions and free accounts of feelings. This particular study aimed to explore and elucidate people's progress, so it was decided to rely on observed weekly changes assessed by the same interviewer and compare different occasions or different groups. This choice means that the 'absolute' values are questionable (when are they not).

Hinton is so committed to the ideal of producing quantitative data that he persists in doing so, despite being aware of and acknowledging these major shortcomings in his method.

In a paper on dignity dialogues at the end of life, Laura Hawryluck use a title which expresses very succinctly our view of the error of attempting to turn quality of life judgements into numbers. She entitles her paper 'Lost in translation' and this is precisely what happens to the attempt to express quality of life judgements in numbers. She asserts that 'concepts of dignity are value-laden, frequently biased, and risk being lost in translation without a deeper exploration of assigned meaning'.[29] We shall discuss dignity in Chapter 3, but simply note here that quality of life judgements are certainly lost in an attempt to translate them into numbers.

2.2.2 Weighting and summing scale items

The simplest way to obtain a final score from a measurement tool is to sum the scores obtained from each item or subset of items. Thus in order to obtain a score for the patient's quality of life one would simply sum the scores from the physical, social, emotional, and symptom domains. However, some items or subsets of items may be more important in quality of life than others. For example, it is possible that freedom from pain and nausea may be more important in quality of life in terminal illness than ability to perform one's social roles. If this is the case then the more important items should contribute more to the overall score. Weighting certain items deemed to be very important is often suggested or carried out. The problem in quality of life scoring is deciding which domains should be given more weight, especially as certain domains will be more important to one individual than another. If quality of life is really just how the individual feels, and a score must represent that individual's value system, then the weighting would have to vary from one individual to another. It is doubtful if such a scoring system could work in practice.

Summing scores from the various domains to obtain a final quality of life score also hides information about the differences in quality between one domain and another. Fallowfield noted this problem in relation to quality of life studies comparing lumpectomy for breast cancer with mastectomy. She notes that several studies showed no difference in quality of life outcomes between the two treatments. She comments that 'The impact that a diagnosis of cancer has on quality of life is not necessarily ameliorated by sparing women the trauma of breast loss'.[30] The reason for the lack of difference in quality of life outcome may be that women who have a mastectomy have more physical trauma due to a larger operation, so that they score worse on the physical domain, but they may have a lower score on anxiety because they may have fewer fears of cancer recurrence. Telling patients that the quality of life outcome of the two treatments is the same does not really give adequate information; patients should be told how the different domains of quality of life are affected by each treatment, since this knowledge is likely to have an impact on their decision.

The presentation of qualitative data by reduction to numbers and statistics can hide important information or mislead readers to erroneous conclusions. For example, John Hinton, in his paper on the progress of awareness and acceptance of dying, stated that awareness of dying rose from a mean of 7.6 eight weeks before death to 8.1 at the last available assessment, (paired $t = 2.45$, $P < 0.05$).[31] However, he goes on to say that many individuals did not follow the group's average path in the final two months. Out of 154 scores from 77 patients and their relatives, 72 patients and relatives showed that awareness may follow any direction. This important message is completely lost by focusing only on the mean score which leads to the erroneous conclusion that the average patient or relative increases awareness in the last eight weeks. Hinton goes on to explain that progress in awareness actually increased in only 15 per cent of patients and relatives, and the change in this groups' awareness caused the increased mean score. An important lesson for clinicians from this paper should be that nearly half of the patients and relatives did not increase their awareness of dying despite the increasing evidence of the last eight weeks of life. Unfortunately this message is obfuscated or perhaps completely lost to most readers because of emphasis laid on the rise in mean scores. Understanding of progress in awareness of dying may actually be impeded by presentation of this important qualitative data in a quantitative form.

2.2.3 Utility rating scales

Economists have devised a series of scales which attempt to assign a numerical value to health states and thus to quality of life. Bowling describes these as utility rating scales. Five types of scale have been used, but we will mention only two which are of relevance to palliative care.

The first is a version of a visual analogue scale (VAS) which is a line, usually 10cm long, one end of which represents health or the most desirable state and is scored as 1 and the other end of which is death or least desirable state and is scored 0. The scorer, usually a member of the public and less commonly a patient, marks points on the line corresponding to the desirableness of various health states. Since the distances along the line of the various points is measured to obtain a score between 0 and 1 for each health state it is assumed that results can be presented as an interval scale. Bowling comments that subjects find this method difficult, and it cannot be assumed that in using any VAS the subject is using an interval scale - it might actually be closer to a logarithmic scale. Despite these problems this method has been used to asses global quality of life in patients with advanced cancer, for example metastatic melanoma.[32]

The second and most widely discussed method of assessing health outcomes is the quality adjusted life year (QALY). This method amalgamates in a single figure an assessment of the quality of the patient's life following treatment plus the number of years to be lived in that state following treatment. Members of the public are asked to consider life in various health states and rate the value of that state between 0 and 1. The number of QALYs gained by a health intervention is the number of years gained or spent in the new health state multiplied by the value in terms of quality of life (between 0 and 1) of that state. Since QALYs have been used in discussions regarding resource allocation a more detailed discussion of the moral problems inherent in that use follows in Chapter 8 on the use of quality of life scales.

Bowling comments that none of the utility scales has been tested adequately for reliability or validity, and subjects very rarely have experience of the illness state they are being asked to value. It is difficult to maintain that people who have no experience of an illness state can evaluate that state.[33]

2.2.4 Should quality of life be represented as numerical data?

We have concluded that research data on quality of life is essentially qualitative, not quantitative. Downie and Macnaughton ask whether researchers involved in qualitative research should use numbers to present their findings—they conclude that they should not.[34] There are five problems associated with presenting qualitative data on the entities relevant to quality of life as numerical scores with attached statistical analysis.

Firstly, since we have no shared and coherent concept of quality of life we are not really sure what we are measuring. When people say they are satisfied with life, we cannot say quite what they are satisfied with, and there is no clear concept of happiness or even dignity—the latter being a relevant concept which we shall discuss in Chapter 3.

Secondly, on the ordinal scales which researchers have tried to develop from questionnaires it is difficult to identify discrete points on what is usually a continuum of experience or meaning.

Thirdly, since the scales used are basically ordinal rather than interval they are not amenable to statistical analysis (apart from identifying the median score). Statistical analyses are often carried out on such ordinal data but are misleading. Such analysis is often presented because the researchers believe that only statistical knowledge will be generalizable outside the study context and might therefore be useful in clinical work and worthy of publication.

Fourthly, whether an interviewer is used or the subject fills out his own questionnaire it is possible that the act of thinking about the questions and dwelling upon one's diagnosis, prognosis, mood, social support and physical performance may have an effect on the results. When an interviewer is used, he or she is part of the measurement tool and may have a major effect on the score allotted to the patient's response. As Downie and Macnaughton say in their previously mentioned discussion of scales 'the measurement tool might distort what is being measured'.[35]

Fifthly, the results of a quality of life study in a particular clinic or by a particular team may well be context specific, and care must be exercised in extrapolating from them to other settings. Salisbury et al. make this point in their review of the evidence of the effect of specialist palliative care on quality of life, where they comment that the generally rapid but variable process of the patient's decline makes comparative studies across different settings and models of organization very difficult.[36]

The second question we raised at the beginning of the chapter concerned the possibility of measuring quality of life. We must conclude that research on quality of life is qualitative in nature and as such it cannot be satisfactorily quantified. Therefore it is not generalizable to other clinical settings in the way that quantitative research is. This is not to say that qualitative research in this context is useless. It is important to review the ways in which people are currently attempting to use quality of life tools, and to ask how the relevant qualitative data which we can gain might be useful in those areas.

2.3 Decision-making for individual patients

Our third queston was whether quality of life questionnaires might help patients with their decisions. Fallowfield suggests that filling in a quality of life questionnaire might aid in the process of choosing the best treatment or management with the patient.[37] She considers that this use of the measurement tools produces few problems. Quality of life assessment might help in clinical decision making in two ways. Firstly, knowledge about the impact of various treatments on the domains of quality of life would help patients, together with their health care team, to make better informed treatment choices. Secondly, it is possible that quality of life assessments might enable better identification of physical, psychological, emotional or social problems in the individual patient.

With regard to the first possibility it seems plausible that qualitative research on the effects of treatments and services on the various domains of quality of life would serve to inform people's choices. The results of qualitative research would be helpful in the clinical context (and would be more helpful than invalid results of quantitative research). Of course, clinicians would always have to exercise judgement in applying the information from such studies to an individual patient—but this is also true of the generalization of results from quantitative studies.

Fallowfield considers that future research and measurement techniques might tell us 'about the changes in quality of life variables which might cause any given patient to accept or reject a particular treatment'.[38] It is inconceivable that any statistical result from quality of life scales could possibly tell us which patients might accept a particular treatment. Moreover, even if such a predictive power were demonstrated, the moral and legal requirements for discussion of all suitable treatment options and for informed consent would remain, so that it is difficult to see how any such predictive power would be helpful either to patients or their doctors. Assuming that quantitative results from quality of life scales could predict patients' choices is analogous to assuming that knowledge of average life expectancy from a given cancer will reliably inform us how long a particular patient will live!

With regard to the second possibility, it seems that clinicians are increasingly convinced that the use of questionnaires or structured interviews relating to the domains of quality of life is the best way to identify patients' physical symptoms, emotional and social problems, and psychiatric morbidity. We have already noted in Section 2.2 that writers in the *OTPM* consider that the lack of use of HRQOL measures contributes to doctors' and nurses' failure to recognize symptoms. But the use of questionnaires and structured interviews is precisely what David Roy in an important editorial has called the use of 'mechanical or instrumental reason'.[39] What is involved is an intervention from outside the patient's own discourse, the imposition of a template on the patient's responses.

This method of assessment contrasts with the traditional method of taking a history, listening carefully, and asking some open questions. The traditional method allows the patient much more freedom of expression and ability to communicate what he or she feels is important than does a questionnaire. The traditional method is also closer to the Asklepian attention, or the listening and watching recommended by Cicely Saunders.[40] Of course, taking the traditional history takes time and can be frustrating for the doctor or nurse, especially when the patient persists in mentioning or dwelling upon aspects of the story which appear irrelevant to the professional.

We suspect that the enthusiasm for measurement tools may be based partly on the idea that they are more cost-effective in that they obtain the answers the professional seeks in the minimum of time, and partly for the less good reason that they place the professional firmly in control of the interaction. It is ironic that workers in specialist palliative care, who have long been advocating a 'patient-centred' approach, should show enthusiasm for methods which are very 'professional-centred'. It should also be noted that the trend towards structured interviews and questionnaires runs completely contrary to the ideal of the patients relating their own narratives, and to the associated ideas of narrative-based medicine. In other words, this trend illustrates one of our central themes: that the Asklepian strand in palliative care, the strand which emphasizes listening and attending to the patient, has been swamped by the Hippocratic strand, which emphasizes interventions and professional techniques and generalizability.

Some examples of papers published in *Palliative Medicine* in 1999 illustrate the growing enthusiasm for tool-based diagnosis as opposed to traditional history taking and allowing the patient to tell the story.

For example, Peter Le Fevre *et al.* published their paper on 'Screening for psychiatric illness in the palliative care inpatient setting: a comparison between the Hospital Anxiety and Depression Scale and the General Health Questionnaire—12'.[41] In this study, they compared the performance of the two questionnaires against the 'gold standard' of a semi-structured psychiatric interview. They concluded that the Hospital Anxiety and Depression Scale (HADS) 'was found to be an effective screening tool' with acceptable sensitivity and specificity. They suggest that the HADS should be used to confirm a diagnosis of anxiety or depression, and furthermore that 'the provision of a validated screening tool opens the door for future "treatment validation" studies'. This latter comment suggests that they consider that a study to assess the outcome of a treatment cannot be carried out unless there is a tool to confirm the original diagnosis. Whilst this is plausible in the case of physical examinations to diagnose a physical pathology, it is less plausible in the context of emotional, psychological or social problems.

Similarly, Peter Maguire *et al.* in 'Physical and psychological needs of patients dying from colo-rectal cancer', reported on the use of a semi-structured interview, a concerns checklist, and the Psychiatric Assessment Schedule to determine patients' physical complaints.[42] They compared the patients' scores with those of their proxies, both informal carers and their GPs, and found poor correlations between the patients' scores and those of the proxies. This group concluded that whilst the use of systematic assessment schedules has been advocated as an effective way of assessing patients' and family problems, 'there is probably no substitute for better training in assessment skills of health care professionals involved in palliative care'. One can only hope that such training emphasizes the importance of allowing the patient to divert from the semi-structure that the professional has imposed on the interview!

Sheila Payne *et al.*, working with the informal carers (usually family members) of patients, used a semi-structured interview and the 'General Health Questionnaire—30' and the 'Carer Strain Index' to assess the psychological distress and strain experienced by carers.[43] They stated that the purpose of this study was 'to identify the perceived support needs of informal carers (family and friends) of cancer patients receiving palliative care in the community'. It is interesting to note that whilst the questionnaires yielded results showing above normal levels of psychological distress and strain, the most informative part of the paper is the section giving direct quotes from the carers' interviews. This section actually allows the reader some insight into what the carers were experiencing. It is difficult to see how a score on a questionnaire could be helpful in comparison with the carer's own description of the problems. The latter information is essential in drawing together possible assistance and solutions, whereas a questionnaire indicating distress and strain is no help in identifying solutions.

Lastly, it should be noted that some questionnaires are highly judgemental in their scoring. This is illustrated in the paper by Ruth Powazki and Declan

Walsh who describe psychosocial assessment of patients and primary care-givers in a specialist palliative care unit using a questionnaire.[44] The purpose of this questionnaire was to identify patients' and caregivers' psychosocial 'needs'.

However, the scoring system in this paper is highly moralistic; a low score was taken to indicate 'high psychosocial risk and need for further intervention, e.g. education and counselling'. Patients would be accorded a low score if they said they indicated they were unaware life was threatened (but some patients actually cope best by not confronting this issue), or if they asked or allowed others to make decisions, or if they avoided conversation with professionals or were regarded as being in denial.

The danger of this sort of questionnaire is that it is identifying some characteristic of the patient as a 'need' for intervention when that intervention is not necessarily a benefit and may even be harmful. Perhaps some patients fare better if they do not acknowledge that life is threatened, if they allow others to make decisions, and if they avoid conversations with professionals. Rather than completing this questionnaire, listening to the patient might have yielded more information about and acceptance of the patient's chosen way of adjusting to the illness and coping with it.

This hazard is illustrated by the 'demoralization scale' referred to earlier in Section 2.2.1. The scale has been developed as the authors feel 'we need a measure that captures reliably its various dimensions and allows these to be followed over time'. They hope that when confirmation of validity is achieved the scale can be used 'as a measure of change in interventions designed to treat demoralization'. Thus this scale has been devised to detect demoralization, since it is assumed that this state is likely to require 'inter-vention' and therefore measurement of it is necessary to ascertain the effectiveness of interventions. We would question firstly whether this natural reaction to the end of life situation actually requires intervention, secondly whether it is in any meaningful sense 'measurable', and thirdly whether the effectiveness of such an intervention can be assessed only by numerical measurement.

With regard to decision-making for individual patients it seems that the hazards of using quantitative questionnaires and structured interviews are likely to outweigh any benefits. The patient's actual description of the situ-ation, or less structured interviews, might best serve to bring to light patients' concerns and point to the possible solutions. Palliative care rightly stresses the importance of being 'patient-centred'. How 'patient-centred' is an interview conducted via a questionnaire (which is necessariy structured), or how patient-centred is a semi-structured interview?

'Quality of life' is also sometimes used in decisions regarding the initiation or the continuation of life-prolonging treatment. Health care professionals tend to think that judgements about the patient's quality of life ought to form the basis of decisions regarding the treatment which should be offered or given. Since there is such confusion about the concept, and there are inherent problems regarding one person judging the quality of life of another person, the judgement of the quality of life of the patient is arguably a very poor basis for decisions regarding provision of lfe-prolonging treatment. In Chapter 5 we shall argue that the soundest basis for such decisions is the balance of benefit to harm and risk. We stress here that judgements of the patient's global quality of life should be avoided in such decisions. Instead, attention should be given to the actual separate effects of the treatment on the length of life, symptoms, function such as mobility, and psychological well-being in the narrow sense to be discussed in Chapter 7. Attempts should not be made to judge the patient's global quality of life with or without the treatment.

We conclude that quality of life is not a helpful concept on which to base decisions for individual patients.

2.4 Quality of life as the goal of palliative care?

Since there is no shared and coherent concept of quality of life attempts to measure it are bound to fail. Whilst it may be possible to agree about which factors may be important in quality of life, a quantitative assessment of those factors either separately or together is not possible. Quality of life as a global concept should not be used as a goal of palliative care, and it follows that attempts to quantify it should be abandoned. This takes us to the fourth and final question we set ourselves at the beginning of the chapter: what should be the goal or goals of palliative care? In answering this question we shall suggest the direction in which we believe palliative care philosophy should develop— back to its original simplicity!

We suggest that the goals should be: the relief of pain and other symptoms; the maximization of physical functioning; and the provision to patients of the information they seek about their illness, in order to enable them to take part in decisions. We wish to draw attention to the fact that these simple measures are those recommended by the WHO in 2004, on the basis that there is evidence that they improve outcomes for cancer patients.[45] To include as goals 'meaning and fulfilment (existential and spiritual issues)' in the manner of the OTPM and in the manner of the WHO definition of palliative care is unrealistic and liable to make professionals who are specialists in palliative care seem pretentious in the eyes of other health care professionals.

Whilst competent and humane care in these areas might increase self-esteem and life-satisfaction, these states are dependent on many factors which are unrelated to health care and which lie outside the influence of health care professionals. Increasing patients' self-esteem, life-satisfaction, happiness or morale are not appropriate goals for palliative care, even though such care may contribute in some small way to their achievement.

Although health care professionals may come to know patients quite well in the context of the illness those professionals are not actually the patients' friends or family, and cannot substitute for them as a social support for the patient. We shall argue elsewhere (Chapters 4 and 7) that care of the family and psychosocial care should not be put forward as goals of palliative care, even though such care may sometimes be of benefit to the patient.

Specialist palliative care may improve aspects of our patients' lives. We should begin by carrying out more qualitative studies on the areas which are legitimate goals of palliative care, and of health care in general. We can place this recommendation within the broad framework of this study. We have distinguished two strands in the tradition of health care which, with some historical licence, we are calling the Hippocratic and the Asklepian. What we mean by the Hippocratic tradition is the predominantly scientific, technical side to health care. What we mean by the Asklepian tradition is that tradition which stresses the special attention, the gaze, the support of the attending physician. Both have a place in modern health care, and the Hippocratic tradition is and perhaps ought to be the dominant one. But the attempt by those in the Hippocratic tradition to colonize what belongs to the Asklepian tradition has not worked well, especially in palliative care. The whole quality of life movement, and persistent attempts to quantify quality of life, are an inappropriate 'Hippocratization' of something which belongs to the Asklepian tradition, whose aims are actually more truly patient-centred, and more humble. Virgil calls medicine the 'quiet art'.[46] Perhaps in palliative care there has been too much busy-ness, too many intrusive questionnaires, and not enough listening.

2.5 **Conclusions**

1 It is not possible to construct a definition of quality of life from our everyday notions about what it means.
2 Quality of life is multi-factorial, its component factors such as happiness, well-being, choice and social factors are incommensurable, so it is not possible to construct a quality of life scale.
3 Research data on quality of life is essentially qualitative and not quantitative—it cannot be rendered quantitative.

4 The quantitative and global assessment of quality of life should be abandoned, and global quality of life should be abandoned as an aim of palliative care.

5 The hazards of using quantitative questionnaires and structured interviews for individual patients (instead of listening to the patient's freehand account) outweigh any benefits for those patients.

6 The aims of palliative care should be: the relief of pain and other symptoms; improvement of physical function; and the provision to patients of the information they seek about their illness in order to enable them to take apart in decisions and lessen emotional distress.

References

1 Kaasa, S. and Loge, J.H. (2004). Quality of life in palliative medicine/principles and practice. In: *Oxford textbook of palliative medicine*, 3rd edn, ed. D. Doyle, G. Hanks, N. Cherny, *et al*. Oxford University Press, Oxford: pp. 196–7.

2 Hippocrates [c.430–330 BC] (1983). The science of medicine. In: *Hippocratic writings*, ed. G.E.R. Lloyd. Penguin Books, London: p.140.

3 Kaasa, S. and Loge, J.H. (2004). op. cit. p.198, Table 2.

4 Lloyd-Williams, M., Dennis, M., and Taylor, F. (2004). A prospective study to determine the association between physical symptoms and depression in patients with advanced cancer. *Palliative Medicine*, 18: 558–63.

5 Chochinov, H.M., Hack, T., McClement, S. *et al*. (2002). Dignity in the terminally ill: an empirical model. *Social Science and Medicine*, 54: 433–43.

6 Ryle, G. (1947). *The concept of mind*. Hutchinson's University Library, London.

7 Kaasa, S. and Loge, J.H. (2004). op. cit. p. 199.

8 Fallowfield, L. (1990). *The quality of life: the missing measurement in health care*. Souvenir Press (Educational and Academic), London.

9 Fallowfield, L. (1990). op. cit. p. 20.

10 Kaasa, S. and Loge, J.H. (2004). op. cit. pp.197–207.

11 Campbell, A., Charlesworth, M., Gillet, G., *et al*. (1997). *Medical ethics*. Oxford University Press, Auckland: p. 138.

12 Bowling, A. (1995). *Measuring health: a review of quality of life measurement scales*. Open University Press, Milton Keynes: p. 4.

13 Bowling, A. (1995). op. cit. pp. 1–4.

14 Bowling, A. (1995). op. cit. p. 9.

15 Kaasa, S. and Loge, J.H. (2004). op. cit. p. 197.

16 Saunders, C. (1972). The care of the dying patient and his family. *Contact*, 38: 12–18.

17 Speck, P., Higginson, I., and Addington-Hall, J. (2004). Spiritual needs in health care. *British Medical Journal*, 329: 123–4.

18 Kaasa, S. and Loge, J.H. (2004). op. cit. p. 207.

19 Downie, R.S. and Macnaughton, J. (2000). *Clinical judgement: evidence in practice*. Oxford University Press, Oxford: p. 27.

20 Bowling, A. (1995). op. cit. p. 12.

21 Karnofsky, D.A., Abelmann, W.H., Craver, L.F., *et al*. (1948). The use of nitrogen mustards in the palliative treatment of carcinoma. *Cancer*, 1: 634–56.

22 Downie, R.S. and Macnaughton, J. (2000). op. cit. p. 27.

23 Fallowfield, L. (1990). op. cit. p. 42.

24 Kissane, D.W., Wein, S., Love, A., *et al.* (2004). The Demoralization Scale: a report of its development and preliminary validation. *Journal of Palliative Care*, 20(4): 269–276; p.276.

25 Bowling, A. (1995). op. cit. pp. 13, 19.

26 Downie, R.S. and Macnaughton, J. (2000). op. cit. p. 28.

27 Bowling, A. (1995). op. cit. p. 13.

28 Hinton, J. (1999). The progress and acceptance of dying assessed in cancer patients and their caring relatives. *Palliative Medicine*, 13: 19–35.

29 Hawryluck, L. (2004). Lost in translation. *Journal of Palliative Care*, 20(3): 150–4; p. 154.

30 Fallowfield, L. (1990). op. cit. p. 100.

31 Hinton, J. (1999). op. cit. pp. 19–35.

32 Coates, A., Thomson, G., McLeod, G.R. *et al.* (1993). Prognostic value of QOL scores in a trial of chemotherapy with or without interferon in patients with metastatic malignant melanoma. *European Journal of Cancer*, 29A(12): 1731–4.

33 Bowling, A. (1995). op. cit. p. 20.

34 Downie, R.S. and Macnaughton, J. (2000). op. cit. p. 32.

35 Downie, R.S. and Macnaughton, J. (2000). op. cit. p. 33.

36 Salisbury, C., Bosanquet, N., Wilkinson, E.K. *et al.* (1999). The impact of different models of specialist palliative care on patients' quality of life: a systematic literature review. *Palliative Medicine*, 13(1): 3–17.

37 Fallowfield, L. (1990). op. cit. pp. 70, 108.

38 Fallowfield, L. (1990). op. cit. p. 216.

39 Roy, D. (2004). Palliative care in a technological age. *Journal of Palliative Care*, 20(4): 267–8.

40 Saunders, C. (2003). *Watch with me*. Mortal Press, Sheffield: pp. 1–8.

41 Le Fevre, P., Devereux J., Smith, S. *et al.* (1999). Screening for psychiatric illness in the palliative care inpatient setting: a comparison between the Hospital Anxiety and Depression Scale and the General Health Questionnaire. *Palliative Medicine*, 13(5): 399–407.

42 Maguire, P., Walsh, S., Jeacock, J. *et al.* (1999). Physical and psychological needs of patients dying from colorectal cancer. *Palliative Medicine*, 13(1): 45–50.

43 Payne, S., Smith, P., and Dean, S. (1999). Identifying the concerns of informal carers in palliative care. *Palliative Medicine*, 13(1): 37–44.

44 Powazki, R. and Walsh, D. (1999). Acute care palliative medicine: psycholsocial assessment of patients and primary caregivers. *Palliative Medicine*, 13: 367–74.

45 WHO (2004). *Better palliative care for older people*. WHO, Geneva: p. 32.

46 Virgil [29–19 B.C.] (1956). *Aeneid*. Translated by W.F. Jackson Knight. Penguin, Harmondsworth: 12, 397.

3

Autonomy, dignity, respect, and the patient-centred approach

Introduction

Although 'quality of life' is the central concept in palliative care as depicted in the WHO philosophy there are other concepts which are also much employed in the regulation of the professional-patient relationship. Important among these are some which are used widely in other branches of health care, and more widely in society as a whole, such as autonomy, choice, dignity, and respect. Other concepts are more specific to health care, such as communication, competence, and consent to treatment. Sometimes concepts such as those mentioned are summarized by saying that they all contribute to 'patient-centred' care.

Nevertheless, although most professionals would agree on the importance of all the above concepts, there is little consistency in their use and not much explicit discussion at least of the broader concepts. An exception here is a recent number of a Canadian journal—the *Journal of Palliative Care* (*JPC*)—which was devoted entirely to studies of the concept of dignity.[1] We shall refer to some of these studies later in the chapter in our attempt to clarify the concepts and relate them to end of life care. We shall begin with autonomy.

3.1 Autonomy, dignity, and respect in Kant

The concept of autonomy (from the Greek, meaning 'self' + 'law', or having the capacity to be self-governing) is central to the moral philosophy of Kant. His development of the concept has been the source of liberal ideas of morality from the eighteenth century to the present, and is largely the foundation of political theories of democracy. The key idea in Kant is that moral imperatives (judgements about what we ought to do) derive from our own adoption of universal moral laws which we apply to ourselves and others alike. The ability to be self-governing in this way, Kant calls 'the autonomy of the will'. Moralities whose imperative force does not come from our own will, but from 'outside' the self, Kant calls 'heteronomous'. Examples of heteronomous moralities are those imposed by an external State, or majority social opinion, or a Church, or by our own empirical psychological desires (and here utilitarianism was very much in his sights).

It is worth noting here, although we shall return to the point in several contexts (Chapter 5, Section 5.4, p. 117), that providing a treatment or a service purely because a patient desires it, may or may not be a good thing, but it is the very reverse of what Kant means by respecting a person's autonomy. To be autonomous for Kant is emphatically not to be able to do or have whatever one desires, but rather it is to have the capacity for rational self-governance. In another of his striking analogies, to be autonomous is to be a member of a kingdom of similar autonomous or self-legislating 'ends-in-themselves'.[2]

Granted Kant's core idea it is easy to relate the concepts of respect and dignity to autonomy and to each other, at least in Kantian terms. Since it was Kant's view that it is autonomy or the capacity to be self-governing which makes human beings unique in the scheme of things, or to be grown-up persons, it was an easy step for him to take to the concept of dignity. Those unfortunate individuals who are pushed around in a heteronomous way by others from the outside, or those who have their decisions made for them, lack dignity; but if you are able to make your own autonomous decisions then you exemplify dignity.

It is worth stressing that Kant's views on dignity are the reverse of many claims made in healthcare. For example, to provide a treatment solely on the grounds that the patient (or relative) desires it but which the best evidence suggests will not work is far from respecting the patient's dignity; it is treating the patient as a child to be humoured. Moreover, the doctor who provides such a treatment is not acting as an autonomous or dignified professional but has become merely an agent of the desires of someone else.

If to be truly autonomous or self-governing is to exemplify a true human dignity where does the idea of 'respect' fit in? Respect is basically a special kind of attitude. If we consider the deference which might be thought appropriately directed to someone of great creative ability, or perhaps to a great statesman, then we might say that we are showing an attitude of respect. For instance, if Beethoven were to enter the room then music lovers would feel impelled to stand up or if Nelson Mandela walked in then those present would in various ways show a deference or respect. It was the moral insight of the Enlightenment, perhaps especially the insight of Kant, to suggest that such deference should be extended to persons as such because persons have the capacity to embody moral values such as honesty. In other words, respect is an attitude of deference or reverence directed at persons not just for their gifts or status, but for being the kind of creatures they are—moral beings—or for their dignity as autonomous creatures. This is the idea behind a large number of well known sayings deriving from the eighteenth century. For example, Robert Burns says:

'The rank is but the guinea stamp,
A man's a man for a'that'.[3]

3.2 Developing Kant's ideas: a bad way and a good way

Kant's views have been developed in two ways in health care ethics. The first way involves an unfortunate narrowing of his idea of autonomy, and an unfortunate change in the meaning of 'respect'. In health care ethics, autonomy has been narrowed to mean simply the ability of people to choose whatever they want. In contrast, for Kant autonomy means to be able to stand back from one's immediate interests or desires and to express moral values, or to be self-governing in being able to act in terms of rules which should be valid for all. The core aspect of Kant's account of autonomy has dropped out of health care ethics and the term 'autonomy' is now used to mean more narrowly the ability to choose what one wants—'I want' has eclipsed 'I ought'.

Going along with this unfortunate narrowing of the idea of autonomy there has been an equally unfortunate change in the meaning of the term 'respect'. For Kant, 'respect' means the deference which might be accorded to a high achiever; he sometimes uses the term 'reverence' instead of 'respect'. But, as we have seen, his moral insight is that this attitude should be directed towards all persons equally, to the extent that they can embody moral values. In health care ethics, however, the object of respect has become the patient's self-determination or his/her desires or choices, and to respect a decision seems to be simply to do what the patient wants. Indeed, as we shall see, some writers argue that to respect the dignity of a patient is just to do what the patient wants, regardless of whether it is in their best interests or of its impact on resources for other patients. This seems an unfortunate way to develop Kant's ideas.

There is however a second way in which Kant's ideas can be developed which is more helpful for palliative care and health care more generally. It can reasonably be argued against Kant that he has an unduly narrow view of human nature. He inherits a tradition of dualism from his predecessors in terms of which human beings have both a rational element in their make-up and also a desiring and sentient element. Kant identifies autonomy with our possession of the rational element. For him our rationality is the divine spark which gives us dignity. Now we do not propose here to argue against a dualistic view of human nature, but will simply assert, dogmatically, that a richer and more satisfactory view of human beings emerges if we are depicted as mind-body unities. We have a body which can suffer pain and we have emotions which shape our identities as much as or more than our rationality does. Thus, we are the persons we are because of how we feel about other people, where our loyalties lie, and the kinds of events we fear. Granted the acceptability of this modified view of Kantianism we shall later try to show that it can contribute to a fruitful and positive way of understanding concepts such as autonomy and dignity as they are used in palliative care.

It is important to note that when we are dealing with competent patients the concepts of autonomy and dignity cover the same area, so that when one concept applies the other does also. But, as we shall see, when we speak of very sick or incompetent patients, or even of the dead, we can still use the concept of dignity even when autonomy is no longer applicable. Hence, dignity is a concept with a much wider area of applicability than autonomy, and *the two concepts are different in essence.* In the discussion which follows we shall see emerging what we mentioned above as the unhelpful restriction of the meaning of 'autonomy' to 'self-determination', and of 'respecting' to 'carrying out the patient's wishes, or choices'.

3.3 Truth-telling, information giving, dignity, and autonomy

The concepts of dignity and autonomy lie behind several more specific concepts in health care. The idea of trust has traditionally been important in the doctor-patient relationship, but what did the patient trust the doctor to do? The answer is that the patient trusted the doctor to try to relieve suffering and to prolong life. Nowadays that tradition has expanded so that trust in the doctor requires not only that doctors will do their best to relieve the patient's suffering but will also tell the truth about it. In the present climate the stress is on openness or 'transparency' in all relationships including professional ones.[4] The question arises as to why there has been this shift, and the answer is that the ideas of the patient's dignity and autonomy have moved to the centre of the ethical spectrum, and brought with them an ethos of openness and the obligation to tell the truth in giving information and reaching treatment decisions. In this section we shall discuss the truth-telling aspects of information giving and their impact on autonomy and dignity, and in Section 3.4 we shall discuss the manner in which information giving should flow into patients' decisions to consent to treatment and the role of autonomy and dignity in that context.

To treat patients in accordance with their dignity, or to respect their autonomous natures, requires truth-telling, because otherwise there is the suggestion that the patient is not able to face the truth, that the patient must be protected in case he/she is frightened. To treat an adult in this way is to treat him as a child, to be paternalistic. For example, sometimes patients are given non-beneficial chemotherapy to 'give them hope'. This is an offence against the dignity of the patient and is very patronising. Furthermore, to provide the chemotherapy where there is no realistic chance of disease response is actually to mislead the patient which is morally worse than simply withholding information. We shall discuss the problems around the giving of hope and false hope in more detail later (Chapter 9, Section 9.4, p. 209).

But of course the patient's dignity or autonomous nature is only one of the factors in truth-telling and the communication of information. Patients in palliative care are approaching the end of their lives so information to be communicated will inevitably be distressing or at least sad. Even if we agree that we must tell the truth, there remain important questions about how much of the truth should be told, how it should be told, and when it should be told. Moreover, the patients will typically be weak and frail and sometimes confused, hence special consideration is necessary to ensure that the information which is provided is understood.

There are two approaches which can be taken to the question of how much of the truth the dignity of the patient requires. Firstly, there is the position that respect for patients' dignity requires that they be told all the information they can comprehend. Secondly, there is the view that since respecting a patient's dignity is only one of the ethical factors involved, the professional's task is limited to giving only that amount of information which patients indicate they want. Of course, if patients are to participate in decisions it may be necessary to give them more information than they want, although less than they could comprehend.

The first proposal can clearly have adverse outcomes, for it means that patients will be given a large amount of bad news, including about likely ways in which they will die. Even if information of this kind is delivered in the best possible manner it may have the result that patients will be unnecessarily traumatized. This is especially unjustifiable when we remember that some of the information may turn out in the end to be irrelevant. The likely adverse effects of this proposal may seem too high a price to pay for respecting dignity in this way.

The second proposal is that professionals should answer patients' questions truthfully but always literally and should not go beyond what the patient is asking. This approach has the advantage that patients can gain knowledge at a pace which enables them to assimilate it. This approach seems to offer dignity coupled with a certain kindness, but it has two major drawbacks.

Firstly, it can be used by the professional as a way of avoiding the responsibility for deciding what aspects of the truth should be told. The professional may be fully aware that the patient's questions may not be leading to the crux of the matter, either because the patient does not know what to ask or is afraid to ask the hard question. Perhaps the duty of the professional who takes seriously the idea of the patient's dignity is to assist the patient in confronting the truth which he suspects but does not quite know how to ask.

Secondly, even if a patient has indicated that they do not want to hear bad news, it may still be the duty of the professional to provide a limited amount of this bad news to prevent further harm. For instance, if a patient with carcinoma of the breast and also neck pain is found to have metastases in the cervical spine, with a risk of cord compression and quadriplegia, then a hard collar should be worn and the patient told to avoid falls. In this situation the patient has to be given the bad news of cervical metastases in order to adjust life style patterns to minimize the risk of the very serious harm of quadriplegia. Clearly, further discussion about radiotherapy will follow, and the patient will need to be told about metastases to consent to this.

Of course, it might be argued that if the patient gives signs that bad news is emphatically not wanted then the professional should not give it—and just hope that the adverse consequences will not happen—but this seems an abdication of responsibility. The other possibility in this situation is to ask permission of the patient to make the best decisions on her behalf without full explanation. The professional can then give advice on lifestyle changes and so on without unwanted explanations of their necessity. If a patient seems resistant to a full explanation this may be the best solution. However, given that the patient will be required to consent to or refuse the radiotherapy, it could be argued that the patient requires the information in order to make that choice. In other words, valid consent may not be possible without the 'bad news'. This situation is a consequence of the current emphasis on adequate information as a basis for valid consent.

The position we are approaching then is that respecting a patient's dignity or autonomy (we use the two terms synonymously here) requires that the professional does not tell lies to the patient. But, since respecting dignity is not the only factor, there may be circumstances in which the professional should be 'economical with the truth', as is sometimes said in political circles. For example, a very ill patient may ask if he has two years to live. The professional may have good reason to think that four weeks is a more likely survival time, but saying this might be unnecessarily harsh. The professional might reasonably reply that survival for two years is very unlikely, rather than that it is impossible. This is far from being the whole truth, but it is truth tempered with kindness. The conclusion seems to be then that respecting the patient's dignity requires that the professional should always tell the truth, but how much of the truth to tell should be based partly on the patient's wishes, and partly on a judgement regarding the potential harm caused by disclosure of the entire truth. In contrast, misleading or deceiving the patient by giving false information or false hope is an offence against dignity, even when motivated by a desire to foster hope. But it is also true that human beings, as we claimed earlier, are mind-body unities, with feelings, hopes, and fears as well as rationality. It follows that respecting a patient's dignity certainly requires truth-telling but truth-telling in a manner and to an extent which takes account of the totality of the elements in human nature.

So far we have been discussing truth-telling mainly in connection with the diagnosis and prognosis. Slightly different issues arise over truth-telling in the context of treatment decisions. As we have already said, we have so far gone along with Kant's view that dignity and autonomy are two aspects of a single concept. We shall later cast doubt on that, but in the meantime it should be noted that if we move to the idea of truth-telling in treatment decisions we are thinking mainly of the patient as autonomous, as having the capacity to govern what happens to his/her body and mind. The idea of autonomy is often expressed in this context via the more limited concept of consent to and refusal of offered treatment.

3.4 Consent, autonomy, and dignity

Of course, the concept of consent probably entered ethical discourse not via the wider concept of autonomy but via common law ideas of bodily integrity and assault. It is normally reckoned to be an assault on bodily integrity if one person touches another without consent. That idea passed easily into medical ethics. Nevertheless, it is against a background of the wider idea of patient autonomy that consent tends to be discussed, and we shall follow that convention.

It is not difficult to see the connections between the general concepts of dignity and autonomy and the more specific concept of consent. In the course of providing health care it is necessary to examine patients, carry out investigations, and provide treatment. Each of these has a direct effect on the patient's body and mind. Given that people are mind-body unities it follows from the ideas of autonomy and dignity that they should have a right to determine what is done to their bodies. Hence, so long as the patient is able to make such choices consent is necessary if we are to respect autonomy and dignity. It is especially important in palliative care to note that consent is also required before pursuing treatment or interventions, including 'counselling', aimed at alleviating mental distress or suffering.

In the ensuing discussion, in order to avoid repetition, we shall use 'treatment' as a generic term to encompass examination and investigation as well as drug and other treatment measures aimed at enhancing the patient's psychosocial well-being. In the first part of the discussion we have assumed that the patient is competent to give consent. As we shall see, when the patient is no longer competent to make decisions the concepts of autonomy and dignity, linked in much writing on palliative care, move apart.

It follows from the concepts of autonomy and dignity (and also from common law ideas of assault) that to consent is to grant someone permission to do what they would not otherwise have the right to do. But there can be various models of consent, which have bearing in different ways on concepts of dignity and autonomy. Let us review these.

Firstly, *consent as being told what is going to be done* is much too weak a notion. Such behaviour is regarded as paternalistic and is an affront to personal dignity (as well as an assault). Secondly, *consent as simply agreeing or acquiescing* to a treatment proposal may still be too weak an idea to count as consent in a treatment context.

This second point is interesting because it indicates that consent, as the term is used in health care, has become a kind of technical term and has pulled away from ordinary life ideas of consent. If I invite you to join me for a drink after work and you agree, you have consented as far as ordinary ideas go. If you do not show up I have a moderate grievance, and it will not do as an excuse to say, "You didn't inform me whether we were going to drink beer or wine, you did not say how long for or where we would be sitting...". Consent in everyday contexts does not require the spelling out of details, but in health care it has come to do so and hence, information is required. How much information is required is an interesting and much discussed question which is not relevant here. The point here is simply that consent in health care is stronger than agreement or acquiescence; we have a right to know what is happening to our bodies.

But of course there may be a range of treatment or care options which are possible and the dignity-autonomy combination gives us a right to choose among them with help from the physician. This suggests a third idea of *consent as joint investigation*. Consent as a joint investigation with the physician is probably the best model. It combines respect for the patient's dignity and autonomy with respect for the consulting physician's dignity and professional autonomy (an idea frequently overlooked in this kind of discussion). In our opinion the joint investigation model offers the best ethical-medical package for both patient and professional. As Arthur Frank has pointed out: 'People know what dignity is by sharing reactions with others who, because they share similar reactions, are *like us*. [his italics] There is no dignity outside of some people-like-us relationships, and people-like-us-relationships require, among other foundational recognitions, shared recognitions of dignity's maintenance or loss'.[5] Dignity is respected then in joint investigation of the best treatment for this patient.

Nevertheless there is a fourth model of consent which has been gaining ground, and is strongly represented in palliative care writings. This we can call *consent as patient self-determination or choice*. As we will see, the narrow view of autonomy as self-determination and of 'respect' as carrying out the instructions of the patient reappear in this fourth model. We have already expressed our rejection of this development of Kant's terminology, and in what follows we shall demonstrate some of its implications for palliative care.

Sometimes this approach is called consent as 'patient choice', but this is ambiguous. There is no problem about patients choosing among alternative treatment options offered—this is what we are calling consent as 'joint consultation'. However, we are dealing with something quite different when we consider the situation in which patients demand a treatment which the professionals judge is not in their best interests. Examples of such demands might include the demand for the commencement or continuation of life-prolonging treatment, or resuscitation attempts, when the doctor or health team are convinced that the relevant evidence shows that such demands are not in the best interests of the patient, because they are most likely to cause net harm, or that they simply will not succeed.

Now this situation can be analysed from several points of view. We shall consider its impact on professionalism; whether it is a case of consumerism; its relationship to human rights; and its relationship to autonomy and dignity.

3.5 **Professionalism, and consent as patient self-determination**

As far as professional integrity goes it is a plausible argument that a professional ought not to be expected to offer and provide a treatment which in his/her considered opinion will result only in net harm. Indeed, in a landmark judgement in the UK the Court of Appeal considered a case (Re J—a minor—1992) in which a physician had indicated that he would not concur with a family's request to give a dying patient ventilatory treatment if that became necessary to sustain the patient's life. Lord Justice Donaldson stated that 'courts should not require a medical practitioner.... to adopt a course of treatment which in the *bona fide* clinical judgement of the practitioner was contra-indicated'. Lord Justice Balcome went further and wrote that he 'could conceive of no situation where it would be proper to order a doctor to treat a patient in a manner contrary to his or her clinical judgment'.[6] In other words, the Court of Appeal is here supporting the professional autonomy of the doctor.

Despite the plausibility of this defence of the autonomy, dignity, or integrity of the profession however, there have been many critics. In a survey of the literature on the issue, as early as 1993 Paris *et al.* note that doctors will almost always continue treatment if requested by patients or relatives even if they regard it as futile.[7] Moreover, this view was supported by many US ethicists throughout the 1990s. Veatch and Spicer (1992) maintain that a physician is obliged to supply requested treatment even if the request 'deviates intolerably' from established standards, or is in terms of the doctor's judgement 'grossly inappropriate'.[8]

This position, in which professional integrity is eroded by patient self-determination, is increasingly adopted in medical practice, especially in palliative care. It is encouraged by three strands of contemporary culture. The first is consumerism; the second is the doctrine of human rights; and the third is patient-centredness. We shall take them in order.

3.6 Consumerism, patient self-determination, and consent

Suppose an ordinary member of the public wishes to buy a basic computer for writing letters, keeping the household accounts, and booking cheap flights. He is shown a bewildering array of machines, and the retailer selects several models which are roughly fitting for his simple requirements. But then the customer's eye lights on a model displaying a colourful and amusing screensaver and he says he wants that model. Now the shop assistant may well explain that that model is much more complex than is needed for the customer's requirements, and that it is twice as expensive. But if, having listened to the advice, the customer persists because he really likes the colour and the screensaver then the shop has no obligation to refuse the sale. The customer is exercising consumer autonomy, and the shop is respecting it. Such a model of autonomy fits well into a free market economy,

Moreover, such a transaction is perfectly acceptable ethically from the point of view of a free market economy, for there are indeed ethical principles in a market model. Thus, consumers must have *access* to the services or goods they require and a *choice* of the goods or services they require. This will involve *competition* between suppliers, and a fair balance in the market place between supplier and customer. Consumers must also have *adequate information* on the goods and services they require; it must be possible for the customer to obtain *redress* in the event of poor services or goods; and the products or services must be *safe* and subject to regulation to ensure their safety.

It would be possible, we believe, to offer a health care service based on such principles, and increasingly there is a move in that direction and away from an older professionally-based ethic. Indeed, there have been attempts by health care managers and politicians to reclassify patients as 'customers', and the language of the market place has begun to creep into health care discourse. But there are three features which prevent the ethics of the free market replacing the ethics of professionalism at the present time.

Firstly, let us return to our purchaser of the computer and imagine he takes delivery of the machine. He tries for several weeks to master its technical complexities and does not succeed. During the course of this he comes to hate the sight of the screen saver and takes the computer back to the shop. The retailer would be perfectly within his legal (and moral) rights if he were to decline to take it back. He could reasonably point out that he had explained that the machine was not suitable, but that the customer had persisted. In short, the customer bears the responsibility for the purchase made against advice. In health care, however, this is not the case. It is the doctor in charge of the case who bears the legal and moral responsibility for the treatment. In other words, there is not now, and not likely to be in the near future, a true consumerism in health care, because the locus of responsibility is different.

Secondly, it is the purchaser in the market situation who puts his money down. In health care, funding is much more indirect, via a publicly funded or insurance funded system. Again, there is no true consumerism.

The third reason is the most important from the point of view of the present argument. One of the important ethical principles of the free market is that goods and services must be safe. It would be morally and legally wrong if a retailer were to supply to a customer goods and services which he knew to be harmful to the customer. For instance, suppose a car owner takes his car to a garage and asks for certain modifications to be made to the engine which (the customer believes) will enable the car to go much faster. If the proposed modifications would make the car dangerous the garage mechanic will refuse to carry them out whether or not the customer demands to have them, but this is precisely what Veatch and Spicer (and many others) seem to be proposing for the doctor (p. 62). As they say, a doctor is obliged to supply treatment even if the request 'deviates intolerably' from established standards or is 'grossly inappropriate', or in the case of end of life attempts at resuscitation, downright harmful. But the basic ethical principle of all health care is now and always has been *primum non nocere*. Yet many ethicists expect doctors to follow patient self-determination to an extent that is not allowed even in a free market. In a free market consumers are largely protected from harm by the law; it is extraordinary that ethicists and lawyers should think that a similar protection should not be given to patients. This issue is sufficiently important and relevant to be discussed further in Chapter 5 on life prolonging treatment (Section 5.4, p. 117). For these three reasons a consumerist idea of autonomy as patient self-determination does not fit the professional situation.

3.7 Human Rights, consent, and patient self-determination

The doctrine of Human Rights is much appealed to at the present time. It has been claimed that Articles 3 and 8, concerning autonomy and dignity, including the right to die with dignity, create a situation in which doctors are obliged to continue life-prolonging treatment, if the patient requests this. This has been argued in a recent UK case (R (Burke) v. The General Medical Council; see Section 5.4, p. 117). However, the judgement seems quite confused.[†] It turns on the premise that it is for the competent patient to determine what is in his own best interests. Leaving aside the obvious point that we notoriously do not always know our own best interests, we must stress that in the case of a patient there is an essential medical element to 'best interests'. Of this the patient, and, it is worth pointing out, lawyers, have no knowledge or experience. It is certainly true that there is more to our 'best interests' than the medical component and that is why patients are entitled to refuse medical treatment. But in medical matters a judgement on what is appropriate to offer medically seems to be the prerogative of the doctors rather than the patient or the courts. This was the view taken in the case of Re J (1992) (see Section 3.5).

It seems extraordinary that Human Rights should be invoked to require doctors to provide a treatment which is inhumane, degrading, and contrary to human dignity simply because the patient says he wants it. Human Rights, which were introduced to try to assert the rights of those who are arbitrarily killed and abused, are now being used to insist on life-prolonging treatment when the medical evidence suggests that it will either fail, or will lead to a life prolonged in inhuman and degrading circumstances. Clearly, this issue will arise only in wealthy countries. We shall take up some of the issues which arise here in more detail in the next Section and also in Chapter 5, Section 5.4, but we should note here that the above judgement has effectively uncoupled self-

---

[†] The judgement (of the High Court) has in fact now been reversed by the Court of Appeal, and the GMC guidance on end of life treatment—that doctors cannot be required to provide treatment not in the best interests of patients—has been upheld.

determination from dignity by saying that self-determination requires a treatment to be given, if the patient wants it, even if to provide it degrades the patient. This issue will also recur with reference to CPR in Chapter 6.

3.8 Patient-centredness, consent, and self-determination

The final point we wish to consider in this context is the most relevant to palliative care. 'Patient centredness' is a central doctrine in the philosophy of palliative care, and this doctrine is often taken to mean that professionals are obliged to follow the patient's desires – we have called this 'consent as patient self-determination' (Chapter 3, Section 5, p. 61). In this section we shall investigate whether this doctrine necessarily follows from the concepts of autonomy and dignity, or whether it is indeed contrary to these concepts. What we shall find is that the two concepts of autonomy and dignity, which we have so far been running in parallel on a modified Kantian model, begin to pull apart.

Instructive here is a paper by Jocelyn Downie, writing in a special issue of the *Journal of Palliative Care* devoted to a study of dignity.[9] Her argument is very clearly expressed and is to the effect that 'unilateral withholding and withdrawal of potentially life-sustaining treatment is a violation of the strong social commitment to dignity as it is understood and reflected in the law by the Supreme Court of Canada'. We are not competent to comment on the views of the Supreme Court of Canada, but will consider her arguments on their own merits without reference to their magisterial backing. Basically her argument is as follows: treatment requires consent, but consent in a medical context (as we claimed earlier) is a richer notion than might be suggested by common law ideas which restrict it to consent to touching of the body. The richer idea is that of consent as following from self-determination, which she and many others (but not Kant) equate with autonomy. Her argument is that the unilateral withholding or withdrawing of potentially life-sustaining treatment disrespects the human capacity for or right to self-determination. This is 'patient-centredness' in its strongest form.

She sees, of course, that one person's capacity for self-determination must be limited by the fact that we all have such a capacity, and so my actions may have an impact (perhaps literally!) on you. But, as far as withholding and withdrawing treatment go, that consideration (she claims) does not apply. There is a resource issue, but we shall come to her discussion of it later. Her conclusion, then, is that the human capacity for self-determination requires that doctors provide life-sustaining treatment because the patient requests it rather than because it is in the patient's medical interests.

She very fairly considers some arguments against this conclusion, and dismisses them. Two of them are less easily dismissed than she allows. The first of these (the third in her argument) is that '[h]ealth care providers are not required to provide treatment that falls outside the bounds of standard medical practice'.[10] Her reply to this is that physicians do legitimately set medical boundaries (e.g. that antibiotics should not be provided for viral infections even where patients request them) but not moral ones (e.g to determine whether resuscitation is worthwhile). The moral bounds must be established by the patient, their proxy, an advance directive, or by the courts.

The trouble with this argument is its assumption that whether or not resuscitation is 'worthwhile' is a moral and not a medical matter. As we shall see when we discuss resuscitation in more detail (Chapter 6), there is overwhelming medical evidence that for patients with advanced malignant disease and poor performance status where death is foreseen, cardiopulmonary resuscitation simply does not work, and its attempt will cause harm by subjecting the patient to an invasive and undignified procedure.

Of course, the cases which Jocelyn Downie outlines at the start of her article are ones in which the patient or proxy should rightly be offered a choice. In her first example the incompetent woman has left a proxy directive requiring artificial hydration and nutrition. Now if it is a medical fact that these will give her a longer life (as distinct from a longer period of dying) then this is a reasonable request. Even more clearly, in Downie's second example, the patient with advanced motor neurone disease and pneumonia who refuses consent to the withholding of antibiotics is entirely within his rights. It is an entirely rational preference to desire a longer life of suffering than a more immediate if peaceful death. These decisions are moral and not medical. But where there is clear medical evidence that a procedure will not work it should be withheld, regardless of the views of the patient or proxy. As we have already stressed, the fundamental principle of all medical ethics is *primum non nocere* and a doctor who offends against this has given up ethically appropriate practice in favour of 'politically correct' decisions or fear of litigation. The situation is even worse when we discuss it in the context of dignity, but first let us look at another of Downie's arguments.

This argument (her final one) concerns resources. It is sometimes argued that doctors should not provide life-sustaining treatment if the medical benefit is marginal or non-existent on the grounds that this treatment will consume scarce resources which might be better employed. Downie's reply to this is that '[i]t is for society, not physicians, to adjudicate between competing interests'.[11] The weakness of this argument is that it does not distinguish between macro and micro allocation. Certainly it is for society (or more realistically a vote-hungry government) to decide the total health care budget and which medical specialties should be allocated varying resources, but the physician works in a particular context in which resources are settled by hospital management. If the physician decides to keep one patient going on a ventilator with no reasonable prospect of recovery some other patients or potential patients will not have access to that ventilator. In other words, a physician cannot easily escape the micro allocation of resources. Moreover, it must be stressed that, since manpower resources are restricted, the nursing and other technical and human resources required to keep one patient alive but incompetent and with no prospect of recovery, mean that other patients may not receive any or adequate pain relief or general care because resources have been diverted to provide the resource-intensive life-prolonging treatment.

We conclude that the patient's self-determination or autonomy (as that term has come to be used in health care ethics) ought to be limited by the physician's professional integrity (*primum non nocere*) and by the physician's duty to use their allocated resources justly. Physicians have professional responsibilities, an issue discussed further in Chapter 5, Section 5.4.

3.9 **Dignity and self-determination**

How does all this bear on the concept of dignity? For an article intended to be about dignity Jocelyn Downie is rather brief on the concept itself. This may be because the concept, as she says, is 'used in connection with a variety of modifiers including: "human dignity", "innate dignity", "inherent dignity", "basic dignity", "essential dignity", and "individual dignity". It is at times related to privacy, reputation, self-worth, self-image, intrinsic worth, and self-determination'. She notes that for her purposes the important point is that the 'Supreme Court of Canada has firmly embraced, albeit in a non-exhaustive way, the inclusion of the capacity for self-determination in the concept of dignity. Thus, we can legitimately move from non-consensual touching to self-determination to dignity and conclude that the unilateral withholding and withdrawing of potentially life-sustaining treatment is a violation of dignity under Canadian law'.[12]

We do not want to comment further on the medical versus moral issue, but just note in passing that of course 'potentially life-sustaining treatment' ought not to be unilaterally withdrawn. But the question is whether, say, cardiopulmonary resuscitation or artificial nutrition and hydration *are* in fact potentially life-sustaining for a patient receiving end-of-life care. This is a medical rather than a moral question, and the answer seems to be that in very many cases in the palliative care context they have in fact no potential for sustaining life. But the question now is whether, if the patient wishes these treatments, respect for the patient's *dignity* requires that they should be provided.

Three considerations suggest that dignity requires that they emphatically should not be provided. Firstly, let us consider the situation (and we have all been in it!) in which we desperately want to believe something which others know is not the case; or in which we desperately want to possess something which we cannot afford or which is not in our interests to have; or in which we desperately want to be loved by someone who does not love us. The duty of friends in such situations is to try to get us to see our lives or situations realistically as they truly are. This is not always easy because, as the poet T.S. Eliot says, 'Human kind cannot bear very much reality'.[13] Nevertheless, when friends make the effort to get us to see straight they are respecting our dignity.

Of course, sometimes people give up on us, or think that it is kinder to us if we are allowed to persist in our delusion. There is a place for that as well, both in ordinary life and in health care. But whatever its occasional merits the second path, of allowing the person to persist in the delusion, is not that of dignity. In other words, if the physician is to respect the dignity of the patient it becomes a duty to try to get the patient to understand the medical facts. Sometimes of course it is not possible to persuade the patient or the relative, and for the sake of a quiet life, or out of kindness to the patient, or to avoid harassing the patient, or fear of the Supreme Court, the physician may capitulate to the patient's demands. But whatever the motivation it cannot be respect for the patient's dignity, although it could be respect for the patient's self-determination. In other words respect for dignity and respect for self-determination are quite different moral concepts. Each may have moral merit, but the merit is different in each case.

Secondly, and related, there are those who, in every walk of life, shout very loudly, threaten, and bully. Often we give in to this and such people (or patients) get their way. But whatever we are doing we are not respecting their dignity; rather we are treating them as the embarrassed mother treats a child who is shouting loudly for a toy or a sweet in a shop. This is the reverse of respecting the patient's dignity.

Thirdly, and we shall discuss this in more detail later (Chapter 6) some of the allegedly life-sustaining treatments are inhumane and degrading. It is sometimes said that, whatever the evidence, CPR should always be attempted, for the patient has nothing to lose. If it doesn't work, the patient would have been dead anyway. But patients do have something to lose—their dignity! CPR is a highly invasive and violent procedure. It may be worth it in an accident and emergency situation where the prognosis for survival is unclear, but it goes against all the tenets of end-of-life care when irreversible failure of vital organs has been identified. In short, it is undignified.

The conclusion then is that even if patient self-determination requires that life-sustaining treatment should always be attempted (and we do not accept this) it does not follow that it is required by the concept of dignity. We must now face the question of how the concept of dignity should be analysed and what its role is, if any, in the conceptual structure of palliative care.

3.10 **The analysis of dignity**

It will be remembered that it was possible for Kant to identify dignity with autonomy because by 'autonomy' he meant not only that people were self-determining but more importantly they were self-governing; they could act as universal law-makers. In other words, Kant thought that to be autonomous was to be able to stand back from one's immediate desires and consider others as equally members of a kingdom of ends. For Kant dignity consisted in the possession of this ability. There are various problems with Kant's position on this but for present purposes the problem is that he restricts dignity to the ability to exercise rational and universalisable choice.

Yet perhaps it is unfair to Kant, it is to misunderstand his historical context, to say that he 'restricts' dignity to autonomy. The point may rather be that in Kant's historical context towards the end of the eighteenth century Enlightenment he was concentrating on just one element in the wider concept of dignity. It was important to assert the importance of that side of human nature which is represented by a desire for a say in how we are governed, and by a reluctance to be pushed around by external authorities. Kant is thinking here of political and religious authorities, which were the threats to individual liberty at that time, but in the nineteenth century J.S. Mill in his essay *On Liberty* is asserting the liberty of the individual against 'the tyranny of majority opinion'; the external threat is social rather than political.[14]

The general point is that when some aspect of human nature is threatened people reach for one of a range of concepts to defend themselves. Sometimes it is 'freedom', sometimes it is 'human rights', and sometimes it is 'dignity'. We are suggesting then that 'dignity' does not name a property which human beings have, but rather it is a normative term suggesting how human beings should or should not be treated in a given social or individual context. As is noted in the *OTPM* '"dignity" in the dying process is a critical goal of palliative care...[but] there is little empirical research on how this term has been used by patients who are nearing death'.[15] Perhaps it is possible to be a little more precise than the *OTPM* implies although such precision cannot be derived from empirical studies as suggested by Chochinov *et al.*[16] In Arthur

Frank's words, dignity (or indignity) claims must 'stand on' something.[17] Can a foundation be found?

Here we might adapt and extend Daryl Pullman's term 'basic dignity'[18] and say that basic dignity rests on basic human nature. Our contention is that dignity or indignity claims arise when some of the many aspects of basic human nature are being neglected or abused. For Kant the basis of human nature is its autonomy (understandable in his context). But although this is a thin conception of basic human nature we have already argued that it can still ground a large number of dignity or indignity claims relevant to palliative care and more generally. For example, as we have seen, granted that people are rational, self-determining and self-governing, it will be an affront to their dignity to lie to them, to delude them, to fail to consult them, to fail to go along with their *refusal* of life-prolonging treatment, or to contrive to find some way round their advance refusal.

But there are many other aspects of basic human nature as well as rationality. This takes us back to the alternative modification of the Kantian position which we mentioned earlier (Section 3.2). Human beings, we said then, are mind-body unities; they are sentient as well as rational. Human beings have a strong dislike of physical pain, they have a desire to cover their bodies, especially their genital areas, and a desire for privacy when engaged in various bodily functions. Whether these desires are universal or simply enormously widespread is a question we can leave to one side. Certainly they extend well beyond western civilization. It will follow from these widespread human desires that patients waiting in public places for clinicians to see them and clad only in inadequate paper gowns may well claim that their dignity has been violated, or patients who are not brought bedpans in good time may similarly feel that they have been degraded. Paradigmatically, patients who are in 'total pain', like Ivan Illich in Tolstoy's story, are robbed of their dignity.[19]

This side of basic human nature is of course important in palliative care and it is one of the areas in which nurses have an important role. It is also interesting that the importance of this side of basic human nature increases as the patient's capacity for self-determination decreases. The majority of patients in palliative care will be very sick, and at some time incompetent. Yet conceptions of dignified or undignified treatment still apply to them when they are semi-conscious or comatose. Indeed, the idea of 'basic human nature' as a base for claims of dignity or indignity still apply to a dead body. This is a deeply-rooted human idea which can be found at the centre of Sophocles play *Antigone*. In the play Creon, the ruler of a city state, has decreed that the body of Polyneices should be left outside the city walls to be eaten by vultures. His sister, Antigone, argues with Creon, to the effect that there is a higher law, a law of nature, that we can all recognize, which insists that even the dead should be treated with dignity.[20]

Whereas it is reasonably easy to see what constitutes respect for dignity when we are dealing with the rational aspects of human nature (e.g. truth-telling and consent) and also for the bodily function aspects (pain relief and privacy mainly), it is less easy to know what will be considered a dignified treatment of a dead body. Here we can go back to Daryl Pullman's distinction between 'basic dignity' and 'personal dignity', the latter being subjective or peculiar to that individual.[21] Perhaps this idea of 'personal dignity' needs to broadened, for much that may appear 'personal' is likely to be cultural. This will apply especially to the treatment of a body after death, but may also apply to how a patient is examined and by whom. Again, some patients find having to be washed, and more generally the loss of physical independence, undignified. Hence, some patients refuse life-prolonging treatment, such as artificial nutrition and hydration after a severe stroke, in order to avoid becoming and remaining physically dependent on others for physical care.

What kind of complaint is made when an action or lack of it is said to be an offence against dignity? Arthur Frank is helpful here. He draws attention to the fact that there can be a spectrum of complaints in palliative care.[22] For example, a physician may be less than polite to a patient and while this could be seriously upsetting, it is not an offence against dignity. At the other end of the spectrum, a physician might actually assault a patient. This is likely to be taken seriously by all concerned, but it is not an offence against dignity. Frank suggests that 'dignity seems to be useful as a mid-level claim'. Hence, issues of dignity are likely to crop up in contexts in which someone's body and their feelings are in the control of others, as is the case in palliative care. It does not require too much imagination, far less the need to go on a course or to have a dignity measurement scale, to have an awareness as a nurse or a physician of what observing the basic dignity of patients will require. But 'special dignity', the dignity which stems from particular cultural or personal beliefs, does require some actual knowledge.

The concept of dignity can be therefore be understood as follows. Respecting dignity requires certain basic forms of behaviour and treatment which we can all understand because we are all human—our patients are 'like us'. In addition there are certain cultural or personal beliefs which patients may have about how to treat them in a dignified way. We must ask about these. So understood dignity has a modest but definite role in the conceptual framework of palliative care.

There are however a number of limitations in the use of the concept. As Ruth Macklin points out: 'A pervasive problem with the concept of dignity is that it is used to defend and justify diametrically opposed actions or practices'.[23] She cites the example of voluntary euthanasia. In discussions of this both proponents and opponents of voluntary euthanasia sometimes build their case round the concept of dignity. Thus, Pullman cites a Canadian Supreme Court ruling concerning physician-assisted suicide in which the justices on either side invoked human dignity.[24] The moral here may be the one drawn by Frank: that dignity is a mid-level claim, and cannot be used to settle high-level controversies.[25]

We are now in a position to answer various questions about dignity. Can it be defined? If by definition we mean a set of necessary and sufficient conditions then it cannot be defined. In particular it cannot be restricted to the ideas covered by self-determination or autonomy. Rather there are a range of contexts relating to features of our basic human nature where it might be 'in gear' as a concept. If relatives attempt to keep the truth from a patient this is an offence against dignity for it implies that a person is not able to face up to fundamental truths about themselves, and if we are rational, competent adults we have a right to know these fundamental truths. Again, it is an offence against dignity if we are not given a measure of privacy for basic bodily functions, or not given adequate pain relief.

Does dignity stretch beyond these basic contexts? Yes, the concept is to some extent culturally conditioned. It may be difficult from our own intuitions to know what a member of another culture might regard, say, as the dignified care of a body after death. This does not require a questionnaire, but a courteous discussion.

Finally, how far can appeals to dignity settle fundamental controversies? The answer is 'not at all'. Dignity cannot be used as a trump card in an argument. Moreover, appeals to dignity can themselves be trumped by other considerations. For example, claims of justice might require that what a patient regards as dignified treatment be waived to provide some more basic pain relief to other patients. Not all palliative care is carried out in rich western countries.

3.11 Conclusions

1 The origins of the concepts of autonomy, dignity, and respect in the modern world are to be found in the moral philosophy of Kant.

2 Kant is able to tie the concepts together because he has a narrow view of basic human nature as purely rational.

3 But even equating dignity with rationality can ground a number of normative requirements, such as truth-telling, and obtaining consent for treatment.

4 A richer conception of 'basic human nature' will include the human body, its feelings and functions. It will also include hopes and fears since these are aspects of our mind-body unity. This broader conception gives rise to a number of dignity-respecting requirements.

5 Dignity and self-determination are different concepts, although they often run parallel. Respecting the patient's dignity does not entail providing treatments simply because the patient demands them; in order to be justifiable, treatments must always carry a likelihood of conferring net benefit.

References

1 *Journal of Palliative Care,* (2004) 20(4).

2 Kant, I. [1785] (1953). *Groundwork of the metaphysic of morals.* Translated by H.J. Paton Hutchinson's University Library, London: pp. 100–2.

3 Burns, R. [1790] (1970). *A man's a man for a'that.* In: *The Penguin book of Scottish verse,* ed. T. Scott. Penguin Books, London: p.330.

4 Downie, R.S. and Randall, F. (2004). Truth-telling and consent. In: *Oxford textbook of palliative medicine,* 3rd edn, ed. D. Doyle, G. Hanks, N. Cherny, *et al.* Oxford University Press, Oxford: pp. 61–5.

5 Frank, A. (2004). Dignity, dialogue and care. *Journal of Palliative Care,* 20(3): [207–11]; 209.

6 Re J (a minor). (1992). 4 All England Reports, 614. *For discussion see:* Hastings Center Report (1992). *British judges cannot order doctors to treat,* 22(4): 3–4.

7 Paris, J., Schreiber, M., Statter, M. *et al.* (1993). Sounding Board. *New England Journal of Medicine,* 329(5): 354–7.

8 Veatch, R.M. and Spicer, C.M. (1992). Medically futile care: the role of the physician in setting limits. *American Journal of Law and Medicine,* 18: 15–36.

9 Downie, J. (2004). Unilateral withholding and withdrawal of potentially life-sustaining treatment: a violation of dignity under the law of Canada. *Journal of Palliative Care,* 20(3): 143–9.

10 Downie, J. (2004). op. cit. p. 147.

11 Downie, J. (2004). op. cit. p. 147.

12 Downie, J. (2004). op. cit. p. 148.

13 Eliot, T. S. (1942). *Burnt Norton, Four Quartets.* Faber and Faber, London.

14 Mill, J.S. [1859] (1964). *On Liberty.* Fontana, London: p. 129.

15 Breitbart, W., Chochinov, H.M., and Passik, S.D. (2004). Psychiatric symptoms in palliative medicine. In: *Oxford textbook of palliative medicine, op. cit.* pp. 757–8.

16 Chochinov, H.M., Hack, T., McClement, S. *et al.* (2002). Dignity in the terminally ill: an empirical model. *Social Science and Medicine,* 54: 433–43.

17 Frank, A. (2004). op. cit. pp. 207–11.

18 Pullman, D. (2004). Death, dignity and moral nonsense. *Journal of Palliative Care,* 20(3): 171–8.

19 Tolstoy, L. [1886] (1960). *Death of Ivan Illich.* Penguin Classics, London.

20 Sophocles [c. 492 BC] (1954). *Antigone.* Penguin Classics, London.

21 Pullman, D. (2004). op. cit. p. 172.

22 Frank, A. (2004). op. cit. p. 208.
23 Macklin, R. (2003). Dignity is a useless concept. *BMJ*, 327: 1419–20.
24 Pullman, D. (2004). op. cit. p. 171.
25 Frank, A. (2004). op. cit. p. 208.

4

Relatives

Introduction

In stating that the goal of palliative care is 'the best possible quality of life for the patient and family', the WHO's description of palliative care clearly implies that the welfare of the patient's family is the concern of the health care team. Moreover, it is also generally taken to mean the welfare of the family is *as much* their concern as that of the patient. In terms of clinical activity this means that the obligation to improve the relatives' quality of life is as strong as the corresponding obligation to improve the patient's quality of life.

Yet professional codes of conduct for doctors and nurses do not include statements about any obligations to relatives but only obligations to patients. It is clear in such codes that obligations of confidentiality towards patients should override requests from relatives for information about the patient's illness, unless patients give consent to the sharing of that information. These codes are widely accepted by health care professionals in the western world, and are implicitly accepted by the community which funds and uses health care services. Similarly, whilst the law clearly states that health care professionals have a duty of care to patients it does not state that there is a duty of care to the relatives, and it too upholds the interests of patients (versus the relatives) in terms of confidentiality and informed consent, and in decision-making for incompetent patients. For example, when a patient has a myocardial infarction, or would benefit from an operation, members of the health care team consider that their obligations are to the patient, not the relatives.

Nevertheless, despite the concurrence of ethical codes, the law and public opinion that relatives are only peripherally, if at all, the concern of health care professionals, the belief in obligations to relatives is rarely questioned in palliative care. This is shown by statements such as the following, contained in a systematic review of the level of need for palliative care: 'Clearly, palliative care services must address the psychological as well physical symptoms associated with the disease process, not only in the patient, but also in the family units supporting the patient'.[1]

Thus the philosophy of palliative care dictates that the relatives of the patient are also part of the remit of care. They appear to be given equal importance to that of the patient. It is perhaps puzzling that there has been so little discussion of the ethical problems which must then arise when there is a conflict of interest between the patient and family. The question must surely arise as to 'who comes first, patient or family?' when such a conflict occurs. Despite the fact that this question is unavoidable if family and patient are given equal priority, some writers either try to avoid it or write what appear to be conflicting statements on the issue.

For example, experienced clinicians Marilyn Relf, Colin Murray Parkes, and Ann Couldrick, writing on counselling in terminal care and bereavement, appear to take two contradictory positions in the same book. Initially, they note that 'As long as patients are alive their needs will come first, but this does not mean that those of the family should be ignored'.[2] Yet on the next page in relation to family members putting the patient first they say:

> Doctors and nurses often do the same [put the patient first], and the result is that we miss an opportunity to help people to prepare themselves for a major transition in their lives. Does that matter? It certainly does and there is a great deal of evidence, from psychiatric practice and research,[3] that major changes in the family, especially if they involve a loss, are turning points that influence the health and adjustment of family members for years and possibly generations to come.[4]

These eminent authors appear to be arguing that if doctors and nurses put the patient first, they miss the opportunity to help the family. Their statement further implies that if, by putting the patient first, we fail to help the family to prepare, then the major change of loss will have adverse effects on the family's health and adjustments for years, and perhaps on the health and adjustment of succeeding generations. The moral problem with this argument is that it leads to the overall conclusion that not only do health care professionals have obligations to relatives, but also that those obligations might legitimately override obligations to patients in some situations. As we have seen, this position contradicts that of professional codes and health care law. It is rightly an uncomfortable position for professionals to take. Hence we find professionals, as we have just seen, stating in one place that the patient comes first yet in another that the family should come first.

This line of reasoning might also be taken to follow from the additional notes to the definition of palliative care, where the WHO reaffirms its commitment to the welfare of the family (as distinct from the patient) as follows:

> Palliative care integrates the psychological and spiritual aspects of patient care, and offers a support system to help patients live as actively as possible until death. It also offers a support system to help the family cope during the patient's illness and in their

own bereavement. Using a team approach, palliative care addresses the needs of patients and their families, including bereavement counselling if necessary.[5]

Once again, the family are given equal priority to the patient, and perhaps even greater priority in that they are to have a dedicated counselling service available to them after the patient's death, should they be judged to need it. This is a more extensive service than many patients can access!

Not only have specialists in palliative care accepted this philosophy, but they have also advocated its adoption by all health care professionals in the context of palliative care. It has become known as part of 'the palliative care approach', and has been advocated as an essential part of the care of patients who are terminally ill. Indeed, it has been held up as an example of excellent care in context of terminal illness.

Thus 'family-centred care' may be recommended, as opposed to 'patient-centred care', without any acknowledgement or discussion of the conflicts of interest which may occur between patient and family. Parkes *et al.* note:

> the unit of care when someone has a life-threatening illness should be the family (which includes the patient) rather than the patient with other members of the family fitted in if we have the time. This conclusion may seem obvious but it is quite foreign to most people who have been educated in a health care system in which the patient is the focus of care[...].[6]

In other words, they are explicitly suggesting that the focus should be not on the patient, but on the family, with the patient included only in parenthesis! This is a frightening example of ideology—if not fanaticism—driving out ethics, and indeed common sense.

Granted the extreme nature of this ideology, as recommended by the WHO, the *OTPM*, and many writers within palliative care, it is important to consider what kind of justification, if any, it could have. It asserts that not only are there general obligations to relatives—to give advice, be courteous and so on—but that there are specific *therapeutic* obligations to family members of the kind which a doctor has to a patient, and that these therapeutic obligations to family members might sometimes override the therapeutic obligation to the patient. This astonishing ideology involves a radical departure from the central ethical tradition of Western medicine. It therefore requires examination and we shall argue:

- ◆ 4.1—that giving the same priority to the quality of life (or interests) of the family as to that of the patient involves unavoidable conflicts of interest, which are often resolved in ways detrimental to the interests of the weakest party—the patient;
- ◆ 4.2—that bereavement care has been shown to benefit only that minority of relatives who have an abnormal grief reaction; bereavement care delivered

to the majority, who have a normal reaction, may not be of benefit and may indeed be harmful.

- ◆ 4.3—that the attempt to benefit families is resourced at the expense of health benefits to patients, for an opportunity cost is attached to all health care; and
- ◆ 4.4—that there are obligations to the relatives of patients of a non-therapeutic but general kind.

4.1 Patient, family, and conflict of interest

We shall argue in this Section that the attempt to treat relatives' interests on a par with the patient's interests results in at least three conflicts of interest, which often work to the detriment of the patient. These conflicts arise over confidentiality, over the place of care and death, and over the time of death. There is also a conflict over resources, for time spent with relatives cannot be spent with patients, but we shall discuss this in Section 4.3 below.

We acknowledge that emotional care of the relatives may be focused almost exclusively on the family as caregivers, and on measures which will enhance their ability to care for the patient. This is the approach taken in the *OTPM* chapter on the emotional care of the family.[7] Assisting families to care for the patient does not generally pose problems so long as the clear priority for health care professionals is the care of the patient, not the relatives. Whilst it might be claimed that the welfare of the two parties cannot be separated, we shall argue that at least three conflicts of interest frequently and unavoidably arise.

The conflicts or contradictions in the palliative care approach to relatives emerge if we examine the benefits which the relatives are thought to gain. Benefit is closely related to the concept of need. Specialists in palliative care speak of the 'needs' of family members. In discussing the emotional problems of the family Joan T. Panke and Betty R. Ferrell state 'Family intervention is needed to confront the many physical and emotional issues associated with palliative care. Intervention is dependent upon assessment of family function-ing and use of an interdisciplinary team to meet the diverse needs of the family'.[8] In so referring to the needs of the family, specialists are meaning both that there will be certain benefits for the family (and perhaps patient) if those needs are met, and also that there is a moral obligation to try to meet those needs. What are these needs and benefits?

In the *OTPM* it is stated that 'while the patient experiences greater physical symptoms, family caregivers often experience a greater degree of suffering as they observe the patient'.[9] The first benefit then is reduction in the suffering of the family caregivers. The second suggested benefit is the prevention of abnormal bereavement reactions. Both benefits are clearly linked. In the chapter on bereavement in the *OTPM* it is noted in relation to the professional role of support for the grieving process: 'Family-centred care is integral to this supportive process as the family's understanding of the illness and its treatment influences their later adjustment'.[10] Since there are links between the relatives' experience of the patient's terminal illness and their subsequent bereavement we are discussing these two alleged benefits in this Section. Conflicts of interest are involved in both.

If we begin with the relatives' experience of the patient's terminal illness we find that palliative care literature suggests that family members have certain 'needs'. These 'needs' have been studied, and results are quoted by Mary Vachon in her chapter on the emotional care of patient, family and professional in the *OTPM* (1st edn).[11] Vachon accepts the results of a study by Hampe in 1975 which identified eight needs of family members of dying patients: to be with the dying person, to be helpful to the dying person, to receive assurance of the dying person's comfort, to be informed of the dying person's condition, to be informed of impending death, to ventilate emotions, and to receive comfort and support from family members and health care professionals.[12] Vachon comments that in this study only three of the needs were met in more than half the sample.

With reference to this (and other studies), Ilora Finlay, concludes 'These studies suggest that the relatives have very specific needs related to the process of loss[. . .]'.[13] She goes on to say that 'The family members each need information to make decisions about their future and to develop ways to cope and adjust to their loss'. Whilst she notes that this need for information may sometimes conflict with the patient's right to confidentiality, Finlay does not suggest how health care professionals ought to act when this conflict of obligations occurs.

It is widely acknowledged that relatives of patients should be given information about the patient's illness. According to the *OTPM*, family members have the following needs for information pertaining to the disease: information about physical care and comfort measures, what symptoms to expect and how to manage them, treatment regimens, expectations for future care, the patient's emotional response, household management procedures and finances, and community resources.[14] The obvious moral problem is that some family members will want information which the patient does not have (perhaps because the patient has not wanted it), or will want information that the patient does not want them to have.

4.1.1 Conflicts over confidentiality

In the *OTPM* chapter on confidentiality, Neil MacDonald does not discuss the issue of confidentiality in respect of divulging information to the patient's relatives.[15] This is not unusual in texts on confidentiality. However, Lesley Fallowfield in her chapter on communication does note that occasionally patients may ask that their relatives are not told the truth. She describes this as:

> a tricky situation as from an ethical standpoint, if conscious, the patient does have the right of confidentiality [...]. The only real suggestion that can be offered in such circumstances, although this is not based on any empirical evidence, is to try and find out why the patient feels so reluctant to share the knowledge about impending death with their relative.[16]

Doubtless this is well meant, but it can easily become officious probing. What is less often discussed is the much more common problem of the family wanting more information than the patient has, for example regarding the likely length of life remaining. Clearly, giving the relatives this information without the explicit consent of the patient is a breach of confidentiality, but is a breach which is rarely acknowledged or discussed in palliative care. We do not think such a breach can be justified in terms of professional codes or the health care law of western nations. Similar problems arise if the relatives ask about future symptoms or modes of dying, which the patient has not wanted to discuss. Yet if, as according to the philosophy of palliative care, there is an equal duty to the family, then one might be justified in this breach because of a benefit to the family.

The failure to acknowledge the limits imposed on health care professionals by the rules of confidentiality is a clear practical illustration of one consequence of regarding the interests of the patient's relatives as being of equal, and sometimes of even greater importance, than those of the patient. This is the first of the conflicts of interests we have noted.

4.1.2 Conflicts over place of care and death

A second important conflict of interest between patients and their relatives concerns the place of care for the patient. Patients may wish to remain at home, but their relatives may be unwilling or feel unable to care for them there. In some cases relatives do not want the patient to die at home because they feel reluctant or unable to live in the house where the patient has died. Less frequently, patients want to remain in hospital or residential care where they feel safe but their relatives want them to be at home. Where a conflict of interests exists it is highly questionable whether professionals should remain impartial on the grounds that they have equal responsibilities towards the patients and their families in terms of enhancing quality of life.

The WHO in its recent document, *Palliative care: the solid facts*, has noted that between 50 and 70 per cent of people receiving care for a serious illness say they would prefer home care at the end of life (although they add that as they approach death some of this group come to prefer inpatient care). The WHO clearly considers that when patients wish to be cared for and die at home, professionals should endeavour to grant this wish. Indeed, it goes so far as to state that: 'Policy-makers should encourage the health services to inquire of people their preference for place of care and death. Meeting individual preferences should be the ultimate measure of success'.[17] Thus it considers that granting the patient's wishes in terms of place of care and death is of crucial importance in palliative care. The implication is that palliative care has not been successful if *the patients* do not live and die where they wish to live and die, but what importance is to be attributed to the relatives' wishes, if they conflict with those of the patient regarding place of death? We believe that policy-makers and professionals must face the reality of frequent conflicts of interest between patients and families on this issue. It is just not possible in every situation to give equal priority to the wishes of the patient and to those of the relatives.

If it is to be the wishes of the patient regarding place of care and death which are paramount, as opposed to those of their caring relatives, then the quality of life of the family is judged to be less important. Platitudes such as 'the patient is indivisible from the family', and the fiction that good communication will resolve all such conflicts of interest, do not solve the moral problem for professionals. The philosophical statement which places equal importance on improving the quality of life of patients and their families, and established practice and teaching which stresses the importance of the relatives' experience during the illness and its effect on their bereavement, both instruct professionals to promote the interests of the family at least as much, and perhaps more than, the interests of the patient. On the other hand, as we have seen above, more detailed guidance such as that given in the WHO publications *Palliative care: the solid facts* and *Better palliative care for older people* clearly instructs that achieving the patient's goal in this respect is of the highest importance, to the extent that it is itself a measure of success of the entire service. These positions are flatly contradictory.

The WHO is not the only organization presenting professionals with this dilemma. The UK standard setting body, the National Institute for Clinical Excellence (NICE), has stated that an objective of palliative care services is to ensure that 'people's preferences on the location of care are followed, whenever possible'.[18] This implies that professionals should endeavour to enable patients to be cared for where they wish to be. It is clearly the patient's preference which counts here, not that of the family, although it is stated that the family should be 'adequately supported' during the process of the patient's death. Once again, the issue of conflict of interest between patient and family has been completely avoided in this national guidance. NICE has followed WHO's recommendations in making it a standard of care that the patient's preference should be ascertained, and success in meeting that preference should be recorded, as a measure of success of the service.

Later in its guidance, NICE notes that: 'It is recognized, [. . .] that for a variety of reasons, not every family member will be able—or will choose—to adopt a caring role'.[19] It states as an objective that: 'family members' and carers' needs are assessed, acknowledged and addressed'.[20] It acknowledges that some family members will choose not to look after the patient at home. One might interpret this as a 'need' to be relieved of the task of caring for the patient. Addressing that need would often, in practice, mean removing the patient from the home. How is it then possible to meet simultaneously the preference of the patient to remain at home, whilst at the same time respecting the choices and meeting the needs of the family?

4.1.3 Conflicts over time of death

The third conflict of interest arises over the use of measures which may alter the time of death. Medications and other treatment measures may have the potential to prolong the final phase of the illness, and sedation may have the potential to shorten it. Conflict of interest can occur when the relatives' desires regarding such treatment conflict with the interests or desires of the patient.

Sometimes carers want to withhold medication from patients, in the belief that it may shorten life or in order that the patient may be more alert for the benefit of relatives. Experienced professionals working in palliative care may then appear to give priority to the needs of the family, and authoritative texts may imply that one's responsibility in this situation is to the family. Whilst it may seem improbable that health care professionals could knowingly fail to consider the patient's wishes and interests, unfortunately this situation does occur. Indeed, in the *OTPM*'s (1st edn) chapter on domiciliary care, Derek Doyle discusses 'treating the patient for the sake of the relatives'. In this section he considers that doing what is in the interests of the relatives (rather than the patient) may be justified, and in one example he completely fails to mention the factor of the interests of the patient.[21]

In the example given, he states that if a patient develops status epilepticus as a result of cerebral metastases from a recently diagnosed bronchogenic carcinoma, then it is justifiable to commence high doses of dexamethasone 'so that in the following weeks as the doses are gradually reduced, the family may enjoy the patient's final days with him'. Doyle's example omits to mention any consideration of the patient's interests. Instead, he advocates striving for a temporary improvement in the patient's condition (hopefully with a return to consciousness), followed by a slow decline, with the *sole aim* of giving relatives time to come to terms with the patient's death. Clearly, a very temporary revival in an uncertain state of consciousness, followed by a steady decline as practitioners reduce the steroid dose, may not be a benefit to the patient at all! One might argue that the patient's dying is protracted for the sake of the relatives.

Derek Doyle was writing in the first edition of the *OTPM*, but the policy of subordinating the patient's interests to those of the relatives is recommended again in the current edition of the *OTPM*. For example, in a case study David Roy states:

> Efforts to prolong the life of a non-salvageable child can be justified, within reasonable limits, if they contribute to the healing of an endangered family life. Treatments of the most varied sorts are means to ends and the futility of treatments in clinical practice should be judged in terms of how likely it is that any given treatment will obtain the *current clinical goal for this patient now.*[22] [our italics]

The first sentence quoted advocates using the dying child only as a means to the end of the family (and for a period of five months). We find this impossible to justify on any grounds, let alone benefit to the parents and sibling. In complete contradiction, the second sentence quoted advocates that treatment decisions should be based only on how likely it is that the treatment will obtain the clinical goal for the patient! Here is another experienced and sensitive author who, under the influence of the ideology, adopts two positions; the first would be judged unethical according to all the traditions of medicine (except palliative care), and the second flatly contradicts the first.

The presence of the above examples in this textbook illustrates the important clinical implications of considering that there is a therapeutic relationship between the health care professional and the patient's family. The results of considering the relatives as 'secondary patients' are clear. The patient's goals, which may be different from those of the relatives, may be completely ignored in favour of the relatives' goals. Whilst there is not a therapeutic relationship between health care professionals and the patient's family, unfortunately palliative care implies that there is by including as a goal of such care the improvement of quality of life for relatives.

It is possible to argue that the mistaken conviction that there is a special therapeutic relationship between health care practitioners and the relatives of patients may diminish the relatives' distress, although it could not abolish it completely. In particular, the relatives may benefit if their interests are pursued even when they conflict with those of the patient. On the other hand, it is equally possible that relatives may feel guilt in bereavement if they judge that the patient suffered in some way because of the pursuit of their own interests. In such cases their overall distress will not be diminished and may even be increased. So it cannot be concluded that the establishment of a therapeutic relationship between health care professionals and the patient's family will inevitably decrease the relatives' distress. And it is certainly the case that at least three conflicts of interest are involved: over confidentiality, over place of death, and over the prolonging (or in some cases even shortening) of the terminal phase of illness. (We shall discuss a fourth important conflict of interest over resources in Section 4.3, below.)

4.2 **Bereavement care: benefit or harm?**

The WHO's philosophy definition dictates that palliative care will offer the family a support system to help them to cope in their own bereavement, and that using a team approach, palliative care will address the needs of the family, including bereavement counselling if necessary. Thus it appears that palliative care teams must provide bereavement follow up of some sort to all families. This is surprising, given that in the same document the WHO notes that there is very little evidence of the benefit of bereavement therapy.[23]

The WHO's philosophy, in the explanatory notes, states that palliative care 'Offers a support system to help the family cope during the patient's illness and their own bereavement'.[24] It would be possible to spell out exactly what giving support entails, the ethical limits (such as patient confidentiality) to that support, the practical limits, and the limits imposed by a just allocation of scarce resources. Yet no attempt is made to consider such moral limits. Later, in the leaflet, following a review of available evidence, the WHO in 2004 stated that there is relatively little evidence for the predictive power of assessments of the need for support and counselling after bereavement, or for the benefit of individual bereavement support. The WHO acknowledged that these interventions are difficult to evaluate.[25]

Assessment of families in an attempt to recognize those at greater risk of poor outcome, and so to provide care prophylactically and plan future bereavement counselling, is recommended in authoritative texts as a way of preventing bereavement morbidity.[26,27] The assumptions used to justify this assessment are that it will actually enable those at greater risk of abnormal bereavement to be identified, and that there are actually care or treatment measures which will prevent the abnormal grief. We would argue that, in the absence of positive evaluations for benefit to relatives from this kind of intervention, there is no current justification for recommending that families should be 'assessed' and 'treated' in this way, nor for expending scarce resources on so doing.

There may be a benefit from one to one bereavement support, provided that the services services can be targeted to individuals at risk. But this does not mean that there is any justification for setting up services which will follow up *every* bereaved relative. Yet strangely, this is what the WHO's philosophy statement seems to require.

Other bodies of national importance have followed the WHO in setting this requirement. Within the UK, NICE issued guidance in 2004 on *Supportive and palliative care in adults with cancer*, also following a review of the evidence. Its key recommendations state: 'Provider organizations should nominate a lead person to oversee the development and implementation of services that specifically focus on the needs of families and carers during the patient's life and in bereavement, and which reflect cultural sensitivities'.[28] This is a surprising conclusion, given that they, like the WHO, acknowledge that risk assessment tools cannot be relied upon as a predictor of bereavement outcome, and that the 'evidence for one-to-one therapeutic interventions for carers is currently unclear'.[29]

The fact that the WHO, NICE, and similar bodies are recommending the establishment of bereavement services, which will inevitably include assessment and individual support and counselling, in the absence of conclusive evidence of benefit, suggests that the recommendation is based on ideology, rather than proven effectiveness. Indeed, NICE goes further down this ideological route when it recommends that 'terminal care [for the patient] supports the view that it should be seen as part of bereavement care, as carers' levels of emotional distress are affected by the care provided before death'.[30] In other words, the care of the patient should be seen as secondary, or a means to, the care of bereaved relatives. This is a good illustration of the power of the ideology of palliative care. Despite the current focus on patient-centredness, the commitment to improving the family's quality of life has resulted in the welfare of the patient being regarded as secondary to that of the relatives!

Given the uncertainties surrounding the ability to identify family members at risk of abnormal or abnormally severe bereavement reactions, and very limited evidence of benefit from one-to-one bereavement support, it seems impossible to justify either subjecting families to formal assessments of their risk for morbid bereavement outcome, or to justify the resources expended in such assessments or one-to-one bereavement services outside of research projects. The exception would be mental health service provision for the small minority of people who are identified as suffering from a psychiatric disorder consequent on bereavement.

The expenditure of large amounts of human (be they voluntary or professional) and financial resources, without evidence of benefit as a justification, is a serious moral issue in palliative care today. We shall discuss this further in Section 4.3 below. Moreover, the doctrine is that support to the family should be continuous through the illness into bereavement. It is noted in the *OTPM* that if preparatory bereavement counselling is not put in place while the patient lives, relatives may reject it. David Kissane comments that 'Attempts to establish bereavement counselling only after the death meet high rates of defensive avoidance blocking this form of support'.[31] But what are those rejecting bereavement counselling trying to avoid, or to defend themselves against? It might be that they are defending themselves against the intrusion of a service which they do not need, or which might actually harm them rather than benefit them.

Further, Parkes *et al.* note that 'there will always be a substantial minority of us who will need help from outside the family' in bereavement.[32] Similarly, David Kissane, in the *OTPM*, writes:

> While over half the families met in a palliative care setting demonstrate resilience through their family functioning, and do not need particular psychological assistance to achieve an adaptive outcome from bereavement, the remainder have identifiable characteristics predictive of a higher risk of morbid outcome and can be specifically targeted through a preventive model of family care.[33]

But what is the evidence of benefit to the 'substantial minority'? Kissane cites only a study from Raphael in 1977. One wonders if other studies have shown benefit, given that, as we have seen, the WHO considers that there is little evidence of benefit from individual therapy. Kissane argues that when preventive interventions are targeted at those at risk, benefits ensue, whereas when they are broadly offered to a bereaved population regardless of risk, no such benefit is discernible.[34] But clearly, identification of those said to be at risk could be achieved only by subjecting every family to an assessment process. This seems an unjustifiable intrusion into private family affairs, granted the paucity of evidence for benefit.

Certainly, alleviation of emotional distress and avoidance of abnormal bereavement reactions are health-related benefits, since they are both likely to lessen physical and psychiatric morbidity. However, the fictitious therapeutic relationship established between relatives and practitioners by the palliative care philosophy entails that the practitioners strive to achieve goals not related to health for relatives. Indeed, the practitioners are bound by that philosophy to try to achieve for the family 'the best possible quality of life'. This might entail suggesting that they plan a holiday, or make alternative career plans, or take any number of measures which could enhance their lives.

It seems totally unreasonable to suggest that health care practitioners should have an obligation to pursue non-health goals for the relatives of their patients, especially as many of these goals could conflict with the interests of the patients.

Moreover, such is the enthusiasm in palliative care to turn relatives into patients suitable for 'assessment and treatment' that it is not considered that this policy might actually be harmful. The harm might be of several kinds. Firstly, the WHO's philosophy statement suggests that feelings of grief, misery, depression, anger, and loneliness are pathological conditions. They are in fact normal human reactions to the ups and downs of human life, a sorry business at best, which frequently involves emotional pain. The idea that emotional pain is a state which requires assessment, medical treatment or 'counselling' is dehumanizing. It is assuming that the best form of human life should always be one of happiness, and that that state can be brought about or its opposite removed, by some form of expertise. The promotion of this idea is a harm to patients, their families and health care professionals.

In contrast, experienced clinical workers have recognized that bereavement is a normal process and that bereaved people are not 'sick'. Parkes *et al.* note that 'Bereaved people who come to think of themselves as sick easily become dependent on those who adopt the role of therapist'. They further comment that specialized counsellors for bereavement 'need to be aware of the dangers of medicalizing normal life crises'.[35] David Kissane, writing in the *OTPM* on formal interventions in bereavement, comments that 'For the majority, although bereavement is painful, their personal resilience will ensure their normal adaptation. There can, therefore, be no justification for routine intervention as grief is not a disease'.[36]

A second form of harm is the implication that ordinary people are not able to cope with the crises of their lives without professional assistance. This is profoundly patronising and deskilling for society; it treats ordinary people like children who need to be comforted by their nanny. We have already noted that even writers enthusiastic about bereavement care agree that input from outside the family is neither necessary nor helpful to the majority of bereaved people.

Thirdly, there is considerable potential for direct harm to relatives. This may occur through intrusive assessment procedures such as those conducted to assess risk of morbid bereavement outcome. Some authors explicitly warn against this harm.[37] Alternatively, bereavement counselling could itself be intrusive or exhausting. Parkes *et al.* describe seven dimensions of loss which should be covered in a single interview, and which if not spontaneously mentioned by the client should be explored by additional questions.[38]

Fourthly, there is a harm to those working in palliative care. Again, Parkes *et al.* note the possibilities of burn out in professionals who have unreasonable expectations of what they should achieve by psychological care of patients and their families.[39] They also note that specialist palliative care is in danger of becoming a victim of its own success:

> The idealized view of hospice care may satisfy society's need for reassurance that it is possible to take away all of the pain and misery of terminal illness. Unfortunately it leaves the professionals who work in hospices (who may have been attracted to the work by this adulation) with the problem of reconciling expectations with reality. Clearly, any job satisfaction must relate to reasonable rather than idealized expectations and it is important for those who recruit and train staff to work in such settings not to collude with cant.[40]

There is also the possibility that professionals may become deluded by being given the idea that by attending courses they are better able than ordinary people to give comfort to the bereaved. But it is well known, and we shall develop this point in Chapter 7, that people with no pretensions to special expertise—the ward cleaner, for example—can be much better at providing human comfort than the 'trained' bereavement counsellor.

4.3 Cost effectiveness of benefit to relatives

Is the health-related benefit to relatives sufficient to justify the expenditure of resources? It is impossible to answer this question in the absence of research comparing the benefit to relatives with the benefits patients could receive if those resources were devoted instead to patient care.

There is some evidence of reduction in relatives' distress in terms of guilt, dependency, loss of control, despair, numbness, shock, and disbelief when patients were cared for within a hospice programme.[41] Nevertheless, research is needed to evaluate the investment of staff time required to achieve this. In such research it would be necessary to distinguish between time invested by staff to assist the family to care for the patient, and time invested in attempting to reduce the distress of relatives where there is very little or no benefit to the patient, for example where the relatives are not caring for the patient.

We have already noted the lack of evidence for preventative measures prior to bereavement, and even enthusiasts claim that such measures would benefit only the 20 per cent of people likely to develop complicated grief.[42] Research would also be required into the benefits of the various grief therapies recommended for complicated grief, since they are relatively expensive in human and financial terms. What is interesting is that within the field of palliative care there seems no interest in pursuing such research and economic analysis.

Perhaps the benefit to relatives from bereavement counselling has not been compared with the benefit patients might receive from use of the equivalent financial resource for the simple reason that it has proved impossible to prove benefit to relatives at all. We note that in the context of scarce resources, where evidence of benefit is increasingly required in order to secure funding for services, cost effectiveness analyses were not required prior to recommending widespread development of bereavement services. But this is not surprising, given that effectiveness has itself not been conclusively established.

At a very simple level it would be interesting to measure the time spent with relatives, and to work out how many more patients the team could care for if varying proportions of that time were used for patient care. Obviously a comparison of the benefit to relatives and to patients would have to be conducted and considered in parallel.

This work may not have been undertaken because a considerable proportion of the funding for specialist palliative care services (more than 50 per cent in much of the UK), actually comes from charitable sources, not public funding. Where palliative care services are not funded either by taxation or insurance, the benefit derived from resources may be less closely scrutinized. Charitable trusts are able to use their funds in whatever way they consider best.

In the *OTPM* chapter on emotional problems in the family the need for research including cost-benefit analysis for patients and relatives is noted. The authors comment that 'Cost measures are essential in the future restructuring of health care, to establish the benefits of palliative care'.[43] We would agree that further research is needed, but it should be done with an open mind, and not based on an assumption that it will necessarily demonstrate benefits from palliative care, or that those benefits to patients' families will be justified by their cost.

In the absence of evidence it is impossible to make a judgement about whether the health-related benefits to relatives could justify the expenditure of resources which are withdrawn from patient care. However, since it is clear that time spent with relatives is lost to patient care it seems reasonable to argue that excessive time should not be spent with relatives. The resource of time must be rationed between relatives and patients. Where significant time is spent with relatives but the staff numbers are relatively low on a ward, then either the staff will pay the price by working persistently more hours than is reasonable or funded, or patients will pay the price by having less than reasonable care, or by reduced access to care caused by closure of beds.

It may be objected that health care professionals in the course of their clinical work already ration the resource of time between patients, even though they have a therapeutic relationship and associated obligations to each patient. The rationing process entails an obligation to distribute benefit justly, as well as to maximize benefit. This raises the question of whether giving benefit to relatives instead of patients represents a fair distribution of resources. It can and should be argued that patients have a prior claim to health care resources over relatives. So where time is scarce, priority should be given to patients. This is not to say that absolutely no time should be given to relatives, but only that patients ought not to be deprived of care essential for their comfort in order to benefit relatives.

4.4 **The nature and extent of obligations to relatives**

Whilst it may be best to say nothing about our obligations to relatives, the idea that their well-being is part of the specialist's remit is so entrenched that it is very unlikely that a new philosophy statement without any such mention would be accepted. Granted this situation, then the statement about any obligations to relatives must be explicit about the nature of the obligations and their limits.

As we have seen in this Chapter, many writers on palliative care depict relatives as 'secondary patients'. If this view were accepted certain therapeutic obligations of assessment and treatment would follow from this special relationship. But we have rejected this view of relatives and their relationships with professionals. Moreover, we have argued against the desirability of seeing *normal* anxiety and grief as pathological states so we reject the idea that special skills are needed (or indeed that they exist at all). But to leave the matter without further discussion is inhumane, for there is a normal human desire to comfort. Here it might be helpful to draw a distinction between what we have elsewhere called, in *Palliative care ethics* the 'intrinsic' and the 'extrinsic' aims of palliative care.[44]

The intrinsic aim of palliative care, its distinctive contribution to human welfare, is to relieve the suffering of patients and prolong their lives if that is possible and their wish. But because of their unique position and relationship with a given patient professionals are likely also to have been in contact with the family. It is therefore entirely appropriate and fitting, and indeed an obligation, that they should offer words of comfort to the family. They should be 'friendly professionals', an idea we shall develop in Chapter 7, Section 7.2, p. 175. Being a 'friendly professional' is the extrinsic aim of palliative care. It does not require 'expertise', but it does require moral and emotional maturity, and the expression of this professional concern and friendship comprises the first type of general obligation to relations.

Secondly, relatives should be given information and explanation about the illness within the constraints of confidentiality to patients. Moreover they should be given realistic reassurance, encouragement and advice when they are participating in the patient's care. But such support should be given with due regard to the time required and the opportunity cost to patients.

Thirdly, when patients are incompetent the relatives should be asked what they think the patient would have wanted, and if possible, their agreement should be reached with the treatment plan. But the patient's interests should not be significantly compromised in order to reach such agreement.

Fourthly, there are obligations to relatives to warn them about possible harms to themselves. Relatives who are caring for patients at home can run the risk of physical injury through inexpert attempts to lift the patient, for instance.

Thus, we have concluded from the above discussion that obligations to relatives are quite different from those which arise from the special therapeutic relationship between professional and patient. Since obligations to patients are those of a therapeutic relationship then they will normally override obligations to relatives if there is a conflict between the two.

An area of conflict often concerns the desire of relatives to protect patients, as they see it, from the truth of their situation. Astonishingly this over-protective approach has been indirectly endorsed by the *BMJ* in a short case example under the general heading of 'A lesson to be learnt' in which the practice of withholding information from the patient at the request of his wife is recommended. The author says 'A family's wishes should be respected where possible, however difficult that may be'.[45] But the point is not that it is 'difficult' to withhold information from the patient at the relatives' request; it is morally wrong to defer to the relative and keep the patient in the dark unless the patient has requested this.

It is possible to argue that a benefit to relatives could appear large in comparison with a very minor harm or forfeit of a small benefit to the patient. Health care professionals may use this argument to justify pursuing the interests of the assertive relatives at the expense of the often vulnerable and unassertive patient. Clearly, members of the health care team will need to weigh up the nature, magnitude and likelihood of the benefit (or the avoidance of harm) to relatives, against the nature, magnitude and likelihood of the benefit (or avoidance of harm) to the patient, bearing in mind that a special relationship pertains in their bond with the patient, and is absent from their links to the relative. The concepts of a *bond* to the patient but a *link* to the relatives might be useful as a way of using language to remind the professionals of the difference in their relationship between the two.

4.5 **Conclusions**

1 Whereas a special therapeutic relationship, founded on an implicit promise and associated with specific obligations, exists between professionals and patients, there is no special relationship, and no implicit promise, between professionals and the relatives of patients.

2 Improvement in the quality of life of relatives of patients is not an intrinsic aim of palliative care.

3 Pursuing the relatives' interests at the expense of the patient's health interests cannot be justified, even in the palliative care setting.

4 Patients should not be deprived of the care essential for their comfort in order to devote time to relatives. Achieving a benefit for the relatives cannot justify inflicting a harm on the patient.

5 The philosophy of palliative care should not state that the aim is to achieve the best possible quality of life for the relatives of patients.

6 There are obligations to relatives of a general nature: to provide information (subject to constraints of confidentiality); to offer advice on the care of the patient; to behave sensitively in the face of the inevitable family distress.

References

1 Franks, P. J. *et al.* (2000). The level of need for palliative care: a systematic review of the literature. *Palliative Medicine,* **14**: 98.

2 Parkes, C.M., Relf, M., and Couldrick, A. (1996). *Counselling in terminal care and bereavement.* BPS Books, Leicester: p. 6.

3 Parkes, C.M. (1996). *Bereavement: studies of grief in adult life,* 3rd edn. Tavistock, London.

4 Parkes, C.M., Relf, M., and Couldrick, A. (1996). op. cit. p. 7.

5 WHO (2004a). *Palliative care: the solid facts.* WHO, Geneva: p. 14.

6 Parkes, C.M., Relf, M., and Couldrick, A. (1996). op. cit. p. 7.

7 Panke, J.T., Ferrell, B.R. (2004). Emotional problems in the family. In: Oxford textbook of palliative medicine, 3rd edn, ed. D. Doyle, G. Hanks, N. Cherny et al. Oxford University Press, Oxford: pp. 985–992

8 Panke, J.T., Ferrell, B.R. (2004). Emotional problems in the family. In: OTPM op. cit. p. 986.

9 Panke, J.T., Ferrell, B.R. (2004). Emotional problems in the family. In: OTPM op. cit. p. 986.

10 Kissane, D. (2004). Bereavement. In: OTPM op. cit. p. 1137.

11 Vachon, M.L.S. (1993). Emotional problems in palliative medicine: patient, family, and professional. In: *Oxford textbook of palliative medicine,* 1st edn, ed. by Doyle, D., Hanks, G.W.C., and MacDonald, N. Oxford University Press, Oxford: p. 592.

12 Hampe, S.O. (1975). Needs of the grieving spouse in a hospital setting. *Nursing Research,* **24**: 113–19.

13 Finlay, I. (1999). Families as secondary patients. *Palliative Care Today,* **viii**(3): p. 42.

14 Panke, J.T., Ferrell, B.R. (2004). Emotional problems in the family. In: OTPM 3rd edn. op.cit. pp. 987–8.

15 MacDonald, N. (2004). Confidentiality. In: OTPM 3rd edn. op.cit. pp. 58–61.

16 Fallowfield, L. (2004). Communication and palliative medicine. In: OTPM 3rd edn. op.cit. p. 106.

17 **WHO** (2004a). op. cit. p. 17.

18 **NICE** (2004). *Improving supportive and palliative care for adults with cancer.* NICE, London: p. 107.

19 **NICE** (2004). *op. cit.* p. 155.

20 **NICE** (2004). *op. cit.* p. 157.

21 **Doyle, D.** (1993). Domiciliary palliative care. In: *OTPM,* 1st edn op. cit. p. 645.

22 **Roy, D.R.** (2004). Eutnanasia and witholding treatment. In: *OTPM,* 3rd edn op. cit. p. 87.

23 **WHO** (2004b). *Better palliative care for older people.* WHO, Geneva: p. 29.

24 **WHO** (2004b). op. cit. p. 14.

25 **WHO** (2004b). op. cit. pp. 28–9.

26 **Kissane, D.** (2004). Bereavement. In: *OTPM,* 3rd edn op. cit. p. 1141.

27 **Parkes, C.M., Relf, M., and Couldrick, A.** (1996). op. cit. pp. 105–10.

28 **NICE** (2004). op. cit. Recommendation 18, p. 13.

29 **NICE** (2004). op. cit. p. 166.

30 **NICE** (2004). op. cit. p. 165.

31 **Kissane, D.** (2004). Bereavement. In: *OTPM,* 3rd edn op. cit. p. 1142.

32 **Parkes, C.M., Relf, M., and Couldrick, A.** (1996). op. cit. p. 192.

33 **Kissane, D.** (2004). Bereavement. In: *OTPM,* 3rd edn op. cit. p. 1140.

34 **Kissane, D.** (2004). Bereavement. In: *OTPM,* 3rd edn op. cit. p. 1141.

35 **Parkes, C.M., Relf, M., and Couldrick, A.** (1996). op. cit. p. 47.

36 **Kissane, D.** (2004). Bereavement. In: *OTPM,* 3rd edn op. cit. p. 1142.

37 **Parkes, C.M., Relf, M., and Couldrick, A.** (1996). op. cit. p. 106.

38 **Parkes, C.M., Relf, M., and Couldrick, A.** (1996). op. cit. p. 147.

39 **Parkes, C.M., Relf, M., and Couldrick, A.** (1996). op. cit. pp. 32–4.

40 **Parkes, C.M., Relf, M., and Couldrick, A.** (1996). op. cit. p. 46.

41 **Johnston, G. and Abraham, C.** (1995). The WHO objectives for palliative care: to what extent are we achieving them? *Palliative Medicine,* **9**: 130.

42 **Kissane, D.** (2004). Bereavement. In: *OTPM,* 3rd edn op. cit. p. 1142.

43 **Panke, J.T., Ferrell, B.R.** (2004). Emotional problem in the family. In: *OTPM,* 3rd edn op. cit. p. 989.

44 **Randall, F. and Downie, R.** (1999). *Palliative care ethics,* 2nd edn. Oxford University Press, Oxford: pp. 16–25.

45 **Solomon, A.** (1999). A Lesson to be learnt *BMJ,* **319**(23): 1105.

Part 2

Interventions, effectiveness, and cost

5

Control of symptoms and prolongation of life

Introduction

The central aims of all health care are threefold: the relief of pain or other symptoms due to disease, the restoration of function (partially or wholly), and the prolongation of life. In the context of terminal illness few moral problems arise in decisions regarding treatments whose sole aim and outcome is the relief of pain or other symptoms. Likewise, if any bodily function can be restored or assisted, such as mobility or cognition, then the worthwhileness of this will not be disputed.

In contrast, many problems arise in relation to the third aim of health care, the prolongation of life. Whilst in health care there is an underlying presumption in favour of providing life-prolonging treatments, this presumption comes into question when the patient is irreversibly dying. Furthermore, the existence of the presumption in favour of efforts to prolong life appears inconsistent with provision of any treatment which may shorten life, either intentionally or unintentionally. Thus the third aim of health care, that of prolongation of life, becomes very problematic in the context of palliative care. We will mention only briefly the moral issues arising from the first and second aims of health care, and will devote most attention to the issues arising from the third aim, focusing both on treatments which prolong life and on those which may shorten it.

The WHO philosophy is open to criticism regarding its approach to this complex and controversial topic, and further development of this aspect of the philosophy is necessary. We appreciate that it is not possible to address this issue in any meaningful way in the short phrase 'intends neither to hasten nor to prolong death'. If the philosophy statement is to say anything about this area of health care then a longer statement is required. We would argue that more consideration should be given openly to the controversy around this issue, which is central to palliative care, and that any statement made should reflect the importance and complexity of the issue.

In the third edition of the *OTPM* David Roy does discuss the issue of withholding and withdrawing life-prolonging treatment, distinguishing it from euthanasia.[1] We support his position on this distinction, and the arguments he puts forward in defence of his position. However, we do think that this topic merits a more in-depth analysis of the basis of the distinction. This analysis includes discussion of some underlying assumptions, and contemplation of the widespread social consequences of abolishing (via legislation and in health care practice) the distinction between withholding or withdrawing treatment, and euthanasia. David Roy also puts forward the arguments for and against euthanasia. We support his conclusion that the law prohibiting euthanasia, even voluntary euthanasia, should be maintained.[2] Since this issue has been well discussed by him, and extensively in the media and literature on health care ethics, we have not included a comprehensive review of the arguments.

In this Chapter we shall discuss the main aims of health care and their interpretation in the WHO philosophy. As we said, we shall deal only briefly with the first two aims—relieving suffering and improving or assisting function (Section 5.1), and at much greater length with the third aim—prolonging life (Section 5.2), and the connected issue of treatments which may hasten death (Section 5.3).

5.1 Relief of physical symptoms and improvement of function

Unfortunately, most treatments for the relief of pain and other symptoms have side-effects which are harmful and so may cause further symptoms and distress. They may also be associated with risks, particularly when an invasive procedure is undertaken. As symptoms in terminal illness—particularly pain, breathlessness, nausea, and vomiting—may be severe, it is often considered that some harms and risks are worth tolerating in order to relieve the initial symptoms. Moral problems arise when the balance of harm and risk to benefit is either uncertain, as is often the case, or when the harms and risks are high in relation to the potential benefit. In such cases it can be difficult to decide which treatments provide sufficient potential benefit in comparison to their harms and risks to justify offering them to the patient. There can be no rigid rules here—the doctor must exercise clinical judgement.

In view of the inherent uncertainty of judgements relating to symptom control the WHO philosophy statement that palliative care improves the quality of life of patients and their families 'through the prevention and relief of suffering by means of early identification and impeccable assessment and treatment of pain and other symptoms' is over-ambitious.[3] This statement places on professionals, especially doctors, the duty to execute thorough and faultless assessment of physical (and also psychological, social, and spiritual) problems, plus a duty to prevent or relieve those problems. In so doing, it also creates very high expectations of those professionals by the public. We would argue that the goal set by the WHO for professionals is unachievable, and that the expectations generated by the philosophy statement are unrealistic. Setting unachievable goals for one set of people, and promoting unrealistic expectations (which will not be met) in another group of people, is unfair to both and likely to lead to harm for both. There is no corresponding benefit for either group which could justify that harm.

The WHO statement may lead to another harm for patients resulting from the term 'impeccable assessment'. If the adjective 'impeccable' simply reflects the need to pay attention to the patient in the Asklepian sense, then it is not morally problematic. It is in this sense which it seems to be used in the *OTPM* with reference to pain control, in the corresponding chapter in the *OTPM* by Kathleen Foley.[4] However, it may be interpreted as a requirement to pursue meticulously a selection of questionnaires which can then be scored, according to the Hippocratic approach. This would drive health care professionals towards impersonal, potentially intrusive and potentially burdensome methods of assessment.

We would argue that the philosophy of palliative care should stress paying attention to the patient's problems, but that the notion of 'impeccable assessment and treatment' should be dropped, on the grounds that it is unrealistic and likely to lead to harms for both professionals and patients.

We said that the second of the main aims of medicine is to improve function. This aim—important in many branches of medicine such as orthopaedics—is not stressed in palliative care. This may well be because the opportunities to improve function are limited. Nonetheless they sometimes exist even in palliative care, and the fact that patients may die in the very near future is not a reason for denying them technically feasible and relatively safe treatments, to help their eyesight or mobility. If patients are to 'live until they die' they must be offered treatments to improve function, such as cataract surgery and physiotherapy, where the benefits clearly outweigh the harms and risks. In this respect palliative care can set an example to other branches of health care which may ignore these needs when it becomes known that a patient is terminally ill. Sometimes, of course, treatments to improve function may have the incidental effect of prolonging life, for example blood transfusions for anaemic patients. It is the issues surrounding this which will mainly concern us in the next Section.

5.2 **Treatments which may prolong life**

The absence of any mention of the aim of prolonging life from the WHO definition of palliative care is perhaps surprising since this aim is indisputably intrinsic to health care. Instead, a short phrase is included in the explanation section of the WHO definition of palliative care: 'Palliative care [...] intends neither to hasten nor to prolong death'.[5]

The definition refers to prolonging 'death' rather than life. The reference to intention is also important here. It makes explicit the idea that professionals have a moral role and specific responsibilities in palliative care, since it is people who have intentions, and the people concerned here are acting in their professional roles. In the context of that role, they must not intend to hasten death, or to prolong death.

5.2.1 **Prolonging death or prolonging life?**

Whilst the phrase 'prolonging life' is commonly used and is widely understood, the idea described in the phrase 'prolonging death' is much less familiar and quite difficult to understand, for death is something which occurs in an instant. Hence we often refer to 'the moment of death', and a precise time of death is notified. Whereas dying is a process of varying length, death is a distinct event which we rightly understand as occurring at a particular moment. Thus in terms of language usage, it makes little sense to speak of 'prolonging death', for it is hardly conceptually possible to prolong that moment when pulse and respiration ceases and brain function essential for life ends.

It is therefore highly unlikely that the WHO was trying to make us believe that the moment of death could be prolonged, and it seems much more likely that the WHO was referring to the process of dying, rather than the moment of death. So the definition might have said 'intends neither to hasten death nor prolong dying'. This is a simple phrase, so why then was it not stated as such? One answer may be that the term 'dying' was deliberately avoided as it is often a matter of interpretation regarding when someone is deemed to be dying, as compared with 'terminally ill'. So it could be difficult to differentiate between treatments which 'prolong dying', and those which 'prolong life' whilst terminally ill. Indeed, there is a sense in which we are all terminally ill!

The WHO probably wanted to avoid this sort of ambiguity and potential confusion, and has attempted to do so by reference to not intending to prolong death. However, since it does not make sense to speak of 'prolonging death', the result of the WHO strategy is that the definition fails to give any guidance on what professionals should intend with regard to treatments which may make patients live longer in the context of an advanced and terminal illness, whether the potential prolongation of life be months or perhaps days or hours prior to death.

This lack of guidance is unfortunate, since decisions regarding treatment which will prolong life for a short time in the face of terminal illness give rise to much controversy and are the source and the cause of many moral problems in palliative care (plus misunderstandings of palliative care by other branches of health care). Rather than providing any guidance or clarification, the current WHO definition attempts to avoid the entire controversy by reference to the untenable notion of prolonging death. In practice, this phrase will probably be interpreted as meaning that one ought not to prolong that very short phase of life, probably the last few hours or minutes, before the patient's death. But in clinical practice this issue is usually uncontroversial anyway, since very few patients, families or professionals seek to prolong that short period when death is imminent.

The 2002 WHO definition has not given guidance regarding prolonging life prior to that point when death is imminent, but this is an issue which has become more controversial as palliative care has developed as a specialty. In its development the range of practice has broadened and the consensus has moved towards provision of more life prolonging treatments, for example technically simple procedures such as blood transfusions and parenteral fluids.

In the early days of palliative care in the UK, when specialists cared for patients in hospices which were largely independent of the National Health Service, life-prolonging measures such as drips and transfusions were rarely provided. There were three reasons for this. Firstly, such measures were seen as yielding little benefit in the face of inevitable death. Secondly, the technology involved was considered to make death less dignified and to prolong the dying phase of the illness attached to tubes and machines. Thirdly, the provision of such treatment was thought to discourage acceptance of the inevitable approach of death, and acceptance was thought to be the attitude associated with least emotional suffering for the patient (and probably everyone else as well). These reasons follow from what we have termed the Asklepian approach to terminally ill patients.

The WHO definition of 1990 stated that palliative care 'neither postpones nor hastens death'.[6] It effectively expressed the idea, from the early days of specialist palliative care, that life prolonging treatment which would simply postpone death, and which might be said to prolong dying, ought not to be offered and provided. This position was not only controversial, but was also inconsistent with that of health care outside specialist palliative care.

Then, as now, health care professionals looking after terminally ill patients but not coming from a specialist palliative care background remain largely ignorant of and uninfluenced by the palliative care philosophy. They know that it exists, but tend to pay little attention to it. They tend to consider it morally acceptable or even morally required that they should try to prolong life, even when death as a result of the illness is foreseen. Thus they tend to provide a life-prolonging treatment unless it is very clear that in the clinical circumstances its harms far outweigh its expected benefits. In this way a situation has developed where 'generalist' health care professionals looking after terminally ill patients tend to think rather differently from specialists in palliative care, despite the fact that both professional groups are looking after the same cohort of patients. So a patient in a particular set of circumstances is likely to be treated differently by specialist and non-specialist health carers.

It is clearly undesirable for this difference in philosophy and therefore in treatment provision to exist within a single profession and health care service. It matters morally because one set of health care decisions may yield a better process and outcome of care than the other for the patient. It is important to ask whether the philosophy of palliative care leads to a better or worse process and outcome of care for patients. Whilst specialists in palliative care now tend to use more life prolonging techniques than in the early days of the hospice movement, they are still influenced by a philosophy which discourages this practice. The WHO definition of palliative care is one important expression of that philosophy, and possible interpretations of it will continue to influence practice.

If 'intends not to prolong death' is interpreted as meaning 'does not prolong dying' then it is likely to lead to a good outcome for patients. In this sense it would influence health care professionals, patients and their families not to pursue treatments which simply prolong the very end of life when consciousness is likely to be diminishing and disturbance to the patient is likely to be distressing. If non-specialists in palliative care were familiar with and accepted this maxim as part of their philosophy then fewer patients would be subjected to invasive and non-beneficial treatments in a misguided and necessarily unsuccessful attempt to prolong life when death is in fact imminent.

On the other hand if 'does not prolong death' is taken to mean 'does not prolong life' in the context of a terminal illness but prior to the period of imminent death, then two serious consequences would arise. The first is that patients would not be offered treatments to prolong life which could provide overall benefit as compared with harm or risk. For example, tube feeding would not be considered for patients unable to swallow because of motor neurone disease or stroke, and stents to keep the ureters patent would not be considered or offered to patients going into renal failure because of incurable pelvic malignancy. Yet for some patients these treatments could provide significant net benefit in terms of prolongation of life prior to that short period when death is imminent.

The second serious consequence is that patients would not be offered treatments primarily intended to alleviate suffering but with a secondary effect of prolonging life. For example, oesophageal stents inserted to alleviate the symptom of dysphagia (difficulty in swallowing) in patients with cancer of the oesophagus may also prolong life. Palliative care practitioners who believe that they should not intend to prolong life may be less inclined to offer such treatments because their secondary effect is to prolong life. Since the phrase 'prolong death' has no commonly understood meaning, it could possibly be interpreted as implying that one ought not to prolong life prior to foreseen death.

Both of these consequences lead to major adverse outcomes for patients. They constitute sufficient reason for rejecting this aspect of the 2002 WHO philosophy of palliative care, insofar as it dictates that health care professionals must not 'intend to prolong death'. This definition is capable of many inter-pretations simply because the idea of prolonging death is logically untenable. Those reading or hearing the definition will inevitably interpret it in their own diverse ways.

It will always be difficult, in a short definition or philosophy statement on palliative care, to address the issue of life prolonging treatment. If the WHO is going to give any guidance on this issue, it would be preferable to use the phrase 'does not intend to prolong dying', which would be more broadly understood.

However, it would then be necessary to acknowledge the existence of the difficulties which surround describing a period of life before death, (excluding the period of imminent death) as either a period of 'dying' or of 'living'. In his chapter in the *OTPM*, David Roy describes 'considerations which refer to the principles most frequently invoked when decisions about treatment have to be made with or for the dying'.[7] In the case studies he presents the patients are clearly at the end of their illness, and would be described by most experienced clinicians as 'dying'. Nevertheless, controversy regarding life-prolonging treat-ment still arises in the cases studied due to disputes or misunderstandings based on the issue of when a patient should be regarded as irreversibly dying.

Returning to the WHO reference to avoid prolonging 'death', it seems likely that the WHO is describing a philosophy of care which discourages the provision of invasive, distressing and expensive life prolonging technology where it is likely to provide overall harm and risk rather than benefit. But whilst this aim sounds laudable and uncontroversial, it has recently been questioned where life prolonging treatment is concerned. In particular, the role of the health care professional, the 'intentions' of the health care professional, and the nature of their duties, have recently been questioned as we shall see in the ensuing discussion.

5.2.2 **Withholding and withdrawing life-prolonging treatment**

This leaves the question about what should be said in a philosophy of palliative care, and in health care ethics generally, about the provision of life-prolonging treatment in an illness which is terminal but when the patient is not imminently dying. In 1999 the BMA after a process of wide consultation produced a document giving professional guidance on this issue.[8] In this guidance it is clearly stated that:

> The primary goal of medical treatment is to benefit the patient by restoring or maintaining the patient's health as far as possible, maximising benefit and minimising harm. If treatment fails, or ceases, to give a net benefit to the patient (or if the patient has competently refused the treatment), the primary goal of medical treatment cannot be realised and the justification for providing the treatment is removed.[9]

This guidance instructs doctors to weigh up carefully in the particular case the benefits of treatment, in terms or restoring or maintaining health, against the harms and risks of the treatment. They must consider (where possible together with the patient) whether the provision of a life-prolonging treatment would provide a health benefit to the patient which outweighs the harms and risks. We would argue that this simple guidance, laid down at the very end of the twentieth century, should be incorporated into a philosophy of palliative care, and could and should be accepted by all health care professionals.

This guidance is also given by David Roy in the specific context of palliative care. Whilst discussing the issue of artificial nutrition and hydration for patients in the persistent vegetative state, he reminds readers of the ethical necessity of justifying every medical and surgical intervention into the body of the patient. He states that the 'ethically critical question' is not 'Are we justified in *dis*continuing this treatment?' but rather: 'What justification is there for *continuing* this treatment?' This statement is made in the context of the argument that benefit (and futility) should be determined in terms of how likely it is that any given treatment will obtain the current clinical goals for this patient.[10]

There is one area of discussion in which the BMA guidance does not go far enough, but where specialists in palliative care are very aware of difficulties in clinical decision-making. Provision of a life-prolonging treatment may not just enable the patient to live longer—it is also very likely to alter the way in which the patient will die. Patients can die of an illness in more or less pleasant ways. Weighing up the benefits, harms, and risks of a treatment does not just entail the consideration of how long one will live plus the side-effects and risks of that treatment. It should also entail consideration of the mode of dying of the illness, with and without the treatment. Unfortunately this factor is given insufficient attention in the BMA guidance, yet it is a crucial factor for health care professionals and patients in making these decisions. Whilst specialists in palliative care are aware of the importance of this factor few other health care professionals routinely think through the likely illness scenarios with and without the treatment. Sometimes specialists in palliative care are less likely to favour a treatment in a particular case as compared with their non-specialist colleagues for the very good reason that the patient may live longer only to encounter a more distressing terminal phase of illness or death.

For example, providing artificial nutrition and hydration to patients with motor neurone disease will prolong their life. Instead of dying of poor food and fluid intake or aspiration pneumonia due to an impaired swallow, they can continue to live but are very likely to become largely or completely paralysed and unable to speak or swallow, making communication very laborious. Ultimately they will become unable to breathe. When this occurs, provision of non-invasive ventilation can once again prolong their life. They will then live until they develop an overwhelming chest infection. The longer their life is prolonged the more likely it is that they will develop the frontal lobe dementia which is associated with this illness. If this happens they will show personality changes, and strange behaviour. Thus decisions about provision of artificial feeding or ventilation must take into account the future development of the illness and the ways in which the patient is most likely to die.

It is perhaps the awareness that life-prolonging treatment may lead to a more unpleasant course of illness and death that has tended to make specialists in palliative care more reluctant to provide such treatment than their non-specialist colleagues. Life-prolonging treatment can be provided without bringing about a prolonged and undignified death, and it does not necessarily prevent patients from reaching a realistic acceptance of their prognosis. However, the achievement of a mode of life and death considered acceptable by the patient requires consideration of the various illness scenarios and ways of dying, as well as the specific benefits, harms, and risks of the available treatments. Not all patients would be willing to tolerate a discussion of the ways in which they might die. This important point should be stressed in a philosophy of palliative care, and in guidance for professional practice generally.

For most people the mode of dying and the period leading up to it are very important. They often seek what Margaret Battin calls 'The Least Worst Death'. She states that:

> In the current enthusiasm for natural death it is not patient autonomy that dismays physicians. What does dismay them is the way in which respect for patient autonomy can lead to cruel results. The cure for that dismay lies in the realisation that the physician can contribute to the genuine honouring of the patient's autonomy and rights, assuring him or her of "natural death" in the way in which the patient understands it, and still remain within the confines of good medical practice and the law.[11]

Patients cannot achieve what for them is 'the least worst death' which fits into the context of their lives unless health care practitioners consider the illness scenarios and explain these to patients who wish to be so informed. Presenting a list of the benefits, harms, and risks of the specific treatment in the circumstances is simply not enough. At the beginning of his discussion on the provision of life-prolonging treatment in the context of advanced terminal illness, David Roy makes this same point when he states that: 'Decisions having such consequences demand that comprehensive attention be given to patients in their full particularity; that attention is focused on the unique biology, clinical condition, needs, desires, life plans, hopes, sufferings, strengths, vulnerabilities, and limitations of *this* particular person'.[12]

5.3 Treatments which may hasten death

The WHO philosophy states that palliative care 'intends neither to hasten nor to prolong death'. The meaning is clear—health care professionals must not intend to hasten death. What is not clear is whether an act which does hasten death, but without intending that effect, could be justifiable. The WHO philosophy statement says nothing on this most important point. So it gives no guidance as to whether a health care professional, in the context of palliative care, should ever perform an act which may hasten death, even if that is not the intention of the act, the latter being carried out to achieve some other goal such as relief of suffering.

The WHO definition also fails to acknowledge an ambiguity around the concept of causation—the extent to which the term 'hasten' implies that one in some way *causes* the patient's death, as opposed to simply altering the time of death so that it occurs earlier.

Thus there are two questions of vital importance in palliative care which the brief definition by the WHO does not address. Firstly, is it ever permissible for a health care professional to make a decision which may result in earlier death of the patient, when that effect was not intended, and secondly, does the idea of 'hastening' death imply that the professional to some extent causes the death of the patient. These two questions can and do lead to enormous confusion amongst health care professionals and patients. As a result of this confusion it is likely that decisions are made which are not in patients' interests. Unfortunately the same confusion almost totally obfuscates any public debate about the issue of legalizing euthanasia. It is regrettable that the WHO definition of palliative care avoids both of these crucial questions. It does nothing to dispel this confusion and may actually contribute to it. The definition of palliative care could have provided some clarification, albeit at the expense of a longer statement, and it is perhaps regrettable that the re-writing of the definition in 2002 was in effect a missed opportunity to provide this clarification

5.3.1 Not hastening death or not intending to hasten death?

The WHO definition states only that in palliative care one must not intend to hasten death. The WHO is effectively saying that professionals must not perform an act or make a decision with the intention of the patient's death occurring earlier than it otherwise would. This is a position similar to that of the law in many countries—that an intent to cause the death of another person is usually a criminal offence.

What the WHO has not addressed is the more difficult question of whether it is permissible to hasten death, if one did not intend to. This is a vital question for two reasons. Firstly, since human beings are vulnerable and death is normally considered an evil there is a general social prohibition against causing or contributing to the death of another person, whether or not one intends to. Thus one will face legal scrutiny for an action, such as a road traffic accident, which contributed to the person's death even if one did not intend injury to the person. Secondly, since an intrinsic function of health care is normally to strive to prolong life there is a general presumption that in health care in particular it is wrong, or at least negligent, to act so as in fact to cause or contribute to the cause of death. For these two reasons there may be a tendency to assume that in palliative care one must never in fact hasten death, even if hastening death is not intentional.

Unfortunately there are three serious adverse consequences to this inter-pretation: it leads to failure to provide any treatment to alleviate suffering if this may also incidentally shorten life; it is associated with confusion around the difference between not providing life-prolonging treatment and acting so as to cause death or alter the time of death; and it puts forward a totally unattainable goal for health care professionals since many treatments are associated with a risk of death through unexpected side-effects.

These consequences are so adverse as to explain why the WHO has avoided stating that one ought not to hasten the patient's death, and has limited the scope of the statement to a prohibition of *intending to* hasten the patient's death. We would argue that it would have been more helpful to state that while professionals must not *intend* to hasten the death of a patient they may *foresee* it, or at least foresee that this is a possible consequence of the treatment. Unfortunately, the concept of intending as opposed to foreseeing an event is not in itself clear to many people in the context of health care. The difference, and the importance of recognising the difference, is discussed later (Section 5.3.4).

5.3.2 Killing versus letting die: the issue of causation

The ambiguity intrinsic to the concept of 'hastening' death gives rise to major problems concerning the causation of death. As stated above, the idea of hastening death can be taken to imply actually causing or contributing to death as the outcome, or alternatively it may imply simply allowing death to occur as a result of the illness. In the latter case one can be said either not to prolong life or to allow death to occur earlier. Whereas causing the patient's death or contributing substantially to it are commonly regarded as 'killing', allowing death to result from the organ failure consequent upon illness is commonly called 'letting die'. The use of these terms has tended to polarize the whole discussion into crude contrasts between killing and letting die. Unfortunately 'hastening death' could be taken to mean either or both.

Allowing death to occur (letting die) has to be permitted when the burdens and risks of life-prolonging treatment clearly outweigh its benefits, or when the provision of life-prolonging treatment so alters the terminal phase of the illness that a more distressing course occurs. At the same time society needs to maintain its prohibition against killing (murder) in order to protect its members. To achieve these two aims, both the law and professional guidance have to uphold a clear distinction between killing and letting die.

The legal situation is fortunately quite clear. In law an act of killing is murder if one person intended to cause and did cause the death of another. It is prohibited in most cultures, and is severely punished. A charge of murder would be brought against a doctor who intended to cause and did cause the death of a patient. Thus if a doctor 'hastened' death by knowingly administering a lethal injection they would be charged with murder. On the other hand a doctor who withholds or withdraws a life-prolonging treatment from a patient because its burdens and risks outweigh its benefits, or because the patient refuses the treatment, is considered to have allowed a foreseen death to occur from natural causes and is not charged with murder. In this situation letting the patient die is legally permitted.

Unfortunately the moral situation is much less clear than the law. In the clinical context the withholding or withdrawing of life-prolonging technology can be seen as 'hastening death'. For example, in the context of irremediable dysphagia due to recurrent cancer of the oesophagus some might argue that cessation of fluids via a drip is a case of 'bringing death nearer' rather than ceasing to put off inevitable and unavoidable death from the illness. The use of the ambiguous term 'hasten death' in the WHO definition causes patients and professionals to regard withholding or withdrawing a life-prolonging treatment as a decision to either cause or bring forward death, and not simply as a decision to allow death to occur from natural causes.

Whilst the use of ambiguous terms such as 'hasten death' has fuelled confusion, the advent of technology has also unavoidably made the moral distinction between killing and letting die appear very blurred in some cases. There are two reasons for this.

The first reason is to do with understandable and perhaps unavoidable ambiguity around the cause of death in a minority of cases. In such cases it may be argued that the withdrawal of life-prolonging or life-sustaining treatment *causes* the death of the patient. For instance, when life-prolonging treatments such as artificial feeding and hydration are removed from patients in the persistent vegetative state, or artificial ventilation is removed from stable but unconscious ventilator-dependent patients, it is overwhelmingly likely that death will follow, and so some people consider that such withdrawal of life-prolonging treatment actually causes the patient's death. They therefore think that it should be considered morally and legally to be the cause of the patient's death. Legally, causing the death is one of the two conditions for murder.

On the other hand, we would wish to argue that the patient's death is caused by the underlying failure of essential organ function (for example permanent unconsciousness or inability to breathe) which renders the patient incapable of survival without constant life-prolonging treatment. The fundamental cause of death is the patient's condition, not the withdrawal of treatment, which should be regarded as incidental. Death would have been caused by the pathological conditions of the PVS or inability to breathe. The life-support treatments merely prevent on a temporary basis the occurrence of death. Such temporary measures give doctors time to assess the situation and to consider whether the body can resume normal functioning or whether there is reasonable hope of improvement. If in these situations there is no reasonable hope of recovery of consciousness or the ability to breathe, further life-sustaining treatment cannot confer benefit and therefore it is not in the patient's interests to continue it. When it is removed the body's own causality results in death.

If this line of reasoning is rejected and it is considered instead that doctors cause the death of patients when they switch off ventilators or remove artificial nutrition and hydration from patients in the PVS, then it must follow that in all cases where doctors have withheld or withdrawn life-prolonging treatment for any reason they have to some extent caused the patient's death. Since the available array of life-prolonging treatment is so extensive, and since the precise timing of so many patients' deaths is now influenced by decisions to forgo some possible life-prolonging technology, one would have to conclude that doctors actually cause the death of the majority of their terminally ill patients. Surely one would have to conclude that doctors cause the patient's death whenever they discontinue a cardiopulmonary resuscitation attempt. The reason is that technically the doctors could have supported the patient's circulation artificially for some time longer. Similarly, the withholding of antibiotics for pneumonia from patients with a very poor prognosis would also be regarded as tantamount to causing the patients death (if it is thought that antibiotics might have prolonged life). Such a conclusion is deeply counter-intuitive, yet it is the conclusion which must follow if one believes that there is 'no difference' morally (or potentially legally) between withholding/withdrawing a treatment and giving a lethal injection which causes death.

This confused position was presented by A.C. Grayling in an editorial in the *BMJ* (2005). Grayling stated:

> Lawyers and doctors distinguish between withholding and withdrawing treatment with death as the result, and giving treatment that causes death. The first is considered to be permissible in law and ethics, the second is not. But in fact there is no difference between them; for withholding treatment is an act, based on a decision, just as giving treatment is an act, based on a decision.[13]

He concludes here that as both decisions result in acts, and after the act the patient has died, then there is no moral difference between the two acts. This means that withholding and withdrawing a life-prolonging treatment in whatever circumstances is morally the same as giving the patient a lethal injection. But as we have seen the confusion in Grayling's position is twofold. Firstly, he is confused over the idea of causality. The cause of the patient's death is not the withdrawing or the withholding of the treatment, but the underlying organ failure. The fact that B occurs after A does not mean that A caused B. Secondly, Grayling is confused over the justification for medical treatment. A treatment is justifiable if, but only if, it has a reasonable prospect of providing benefit exceeding harm and risk. When that is not the case the treatment ought to be withdrawn or withheld.

Moreover, if doctors were considered to have caused the patient's death whenever they withheld or withdrew life-prolonging treatment the law would have to examine each incident as a possible case of murder. If it were judged that the doctor might have intended the death of the patient (which he or she was considered to have caused) then a charge of murder would have to be made. This situation would be completely unmanageable legally. But if withholding and withdrawing life-prolonging treatment is considered to cause death this unmanageable legal situation could be avoided only if the prohibition against intentionally causing death were abolished. Such an alteration in the law would be highly undesirable because it would remove an essential protection for all members of society.

One must conclude that in health care ethics (including palliative care) and the law, 'letting die' in the sense of withholding or withdrawing non-beneficial life-prolonging treatment must be permitted and even advocated. As the BMA states, if there is no expected net benefit to the patient then there is no justification for providing the treatment.

5.3.3 Intending versus foreseeing death

The second reason for the blurring of the moral distinction between killing and letting die has to do with the distinction between intending and foreseeing the outcome of a decision. The importance of this distinction in respect of the ambiguity around 'not hastening death' was mentioned above (Section 5.3.1). The moral distinction between intending and foreseeing the death of the patient following withholding or withdrawal of life-prolonging treatment may be finely drawn. It is sometimes argued that when a doctor switches off a ventilator-dependent patient's ventilator, or removes artificial feeding and hydration from a patient in the persistent vegetative state, that doctor is intending to cause the patient's death. Once again, this would be the position taken by Grayling. He believes that the distinction drawn between intending and foreseeing an outcome, as in the doctrine of double effect, is 'fictitious'.[14] Those who take this position assert that the doctor must inevitably intend the patient's death since he or she knows that it is overwhelmingly likely that death will follow withdrawal of these treatments. The contrary position, which we hold, is that the doctor intends only to withdraw a futile and non-beneficial treatment, and foresees but does not intend the patient's death.

There are two specific aspects to intention in this case, and a more general point about intending and foreseeing. The first specific point is to do with what the doctor wants, desires or seeks as the outcome of the decision. Some people who maintain that the doctor intends the patient's death seem to believe that the doctor wants or desires the patient's death. Yet this is surely not the most accurate representation of the case. The doctor is in no way seeking the patient's death, even if it is agreed that death is the least bad outcome because it is considered preferable to continued existence in a state of profound disability, distress or discomfort. The representation which we consider most accurately describes the case is that the doctor neither desires nor seeks the patients death, but rather intends only to withdraw or withhold a non-beneficial and possibly burdensome treatment. No doctor should seek a patient's death, but equally no doctor wants (or should want) to impose a treatment which confers no benefit and which may be burdensome.

The second specific point or aspect of intention relates to the fact that it is intention *to cause* the death of the patient which is being considered. Thus those who believe that the doctor who withdraws or withholds life-prolonging treatment intends the patient's death must believe that the doctor intends *to cause* the patient's death. In reply we would argue that since doctors quite reasonably do not consider that the withdrawal or withholding of life-prolonging treatment is the fundamental cause of the patient's death, they cannot logically intend to cause death by withholding or withdrawing treatment. It makes no sense to argue that doctors intend to cause death when they do not think their decision is the cause of that death.

The general point is that there is a clear conceptual distinction between intending and foreseeing. Foreseeing may not be connected with human agency at all—as when a farmer foresees a bad harvest. But even when foreseeing is connected with human agency its connection is oblique and consequential rather than intentional. For example, when a surgeon carries out an operation (an intentional act) he will foresee that the patient will later feel discomfort, but to say that he intends the discomfort is absurd.

In summary, then, we would argue that doctors who withhold or withdraw life-prolonging treatment when its burdens outweigh its benefits do not cause nor intend to cause the patient's death. Rather, they withhold or withdraw treatment which they consider is inappropriate because its burdens exceed its benefits, and they foresee the patient's death but do not desire or seek it, nor intend to cause it. Somehow the philosophy of palliative care, as an integral and consistent part of health care ethics, must succeed in making these distinctions clear to other branches of health care, whilst at the same time continuing to prohibit professionals from intentionally causing the death of their patients.

5.3.4 Double effect

The preceding discussion centres on the possible interpretation of withholding or withdrawing life-prolonging treatment as in some way causing or 'hastening' death. However, there are clinical situations in which a treatment given with the aim of relieving distressing symptoms at the end of life may actually have other effects which may make death occur earlier than it would have done without the treatment. It is important to remember that such treatments are not the cause of death entirely, but in the context of the patient's advanced illness and frailty death may occur earlier than without the treatment. The doctrine of double effect is commonly used to justify the provision of such treatments even though they may 'hasten' death in the sense of bringing it forward. One must ask whether this doctrine is essential or even useful in the philosophy of palliative care, and whether there is any alternative professional guidance which would lead to better decisions.

It is important to note that the circumstances in which the only way to alleviate pain or distress is to use a treatment which may bring forward death are really quite rare. There is a common misconception that morphine will shorten life by causing respiratory depression and sedation. Properly used, and used only as an analgesic (not as a sedative), this is not the case. Patients given only the amount of morphine needed to counterbalance and relieve a morphine-sensitive pain do not suffer respiratory depression and are not sedated. Thus the example of morphine, which is unfortunately commonly given in the media, is totally misleading and simply causes the public and professionals to maintain fear and reluctance regarding its use.

On the other hand there are circumstances where sedation or sometimes a technical procedure may bring death nearer. Patients who are confused at the end of life may become restless and agitated. Sedation by drugs like diazepam alleviates this distress but if the distress passes only when the patient is rendered very drowsy or asleep then clearly the patient drinks less, moves less, and so may be more likely to develop pneumonia. Similarly, a procedure like paracentesis (removal of abnormal fluid collections from the abdomen) may be the most effective way to alleviate distress due to a very distended abdomen associated with difficulty breathing. However, when the patient is very ill the loss of litres of fluid from the abdominal cavity may precipitate shock and death may occur earlier than if the paracentesis had not been done. These are genuine examples of situations where a treatment intended to alleviate symptoms may cause death to occur earlier, but the treatments are not themselves the primary cause of death. This is brought out if we consider that the same treatments given to a healthier person would not bring about death at all, and death occurs in these patients primarily because of the advanced state of their illness.

The present issue however is whether these important distinctions are best explained via the doctrine of double effect. This doctrine claims that a single act with both good and bad effects is justified *if, and only if,* four conditions are met. It is important to note that all four conditions must be met. The doctrine itself has a long history and is used in a variety of contexts. Many textbooks on ethics discuss the doctrine, but a standard account of the four conditions is provided by Tom L. Beauchamp and James F. Childress in *Principles of biomedical ethics.*[15] The four conditions are:

1 *The nature of the act.* The act must be good, or at least morally neutral (independent of its consequences).
2 *The agent's intention.* The agent intends only the good effect. The bad effect can be foreseen, tolerated, and permitted, but it must not be intended.
3 *The distinction between means and effects.* The bad effect must not be a means to the good effect. If the good effect were the direct causal result of the bad effect, the agent would intend the bad effect in pursuit of the good effect.
4 *Proportionality between the good effect and the bad effect.* The good effect must outweigh the bad effect. The bad effect is permissible only if a proportionate reason is present that compensates for permitting the foreseen bad effect.

It can be seen that decisions to provide a treatment to alleviate distress or pain in the context of terminal illness may sometimes meet all of the above conditions and so be considered permitted according to the doctrine. For example, the nature of the act of providing symptom relief is morally good, the agent might intend only the good effect of relief of distress but not the bad effect of hastening death, the relief of suffering is brought about by the treatment and not by the bad effect which is the earlier death of the patient, and the good of relieving suffering in the face of inevitable death in the near future outweighs the bad effect of hastening that death.

The main problem with the use of the doctrine in health care ethics, even in the specialist field of palliative care, is that many if not most health care professionals are unaware of the four conditions, are unable to understand them, or are unable to remember them. They therefore tend to think that the doctrine means simply that an act with a bad effect, such as the death of the patient, is justified if the agent did not intend the bad effect, even though it was foreseen. This misconception of the doctrine actually leads to its abuse. For example, some people have suggested that euthanasia is justified by the doctrine of double effect, whereas this could never be the case because in euthanasia the bad effect is intended, and the good effect is brought about via the bad effect, so conditions 2 and 3 above are not met. For these reasons the doctrine itself should be rejected as a part of a philosophy of palliative care, even though its proper use might in theory be helpful in clinical practice.

Instead, a philosophy of palliative care as part of a more general health care ethics should make clear that in making decisions practitioners must weigh up carefully the benefits, harms and risks of a treatment in the particular patient's case, and that practitioners must not intentionally cause the patient's death.

Most health care professionals will fully comprehend and use such guidance only if examples in the form of case scenarios are used in education. The methods of casuistry would help practitioners to judge whether provision of a treatment with a foreseen bad effect as well as the intended good effect was justified in particular circumstances.

5.3.5 Euthanasia and letting die

We have stated that the philosophy of palliative care, and health care ethics in general, should continue to prohibit practitioners from intentionally causing the death of their patients. However, since euthanasia is one of the many moral questions on which opinions differ some people will inevitably disagree with us. Those who do sometimes develop an argument to suggest that the legal prohibition of 'mercy killing' should be revoked. (In this context we mean by 'mercy killing' or 'euthanasia' an intentional act which causes the death of the patient and which is done through compassionate motives.) If the legal prohibition of euthanasia were revoked and it were legalized, then clearly the philosophy of palliative care and professional ethics in health care would have to be altered in very significant ways with many important implications. These implications are discussed by David Roy in the *OTPM*, where he argues *against* the legalization of euthanasia.[16]

We will now analyse one particular argument, which is often raised in favour of legalizing euthanasia, but which is rarely studied in sufficient depth. The proponents of euthanasia often argue that there is no significant moral difference between intentionally causing the death of a patient (mercy killing or euthanasia) and withholding or withdrawing life-prolonging treatment (acts fitting our description of letting die). In other words they assert that letting die is morally indistinguishable from euthanasia or mercy killing. (This is the argument quoted above, by A.C. Grayling.) They also assert that the law should treat acts which are considered morally indistinguishable in the same way, so that if letting die is permitted so should acts of mercy killing or euthanasia be permitted. Their arguments can be presented as a logical syllogism as follows:

Major premise: Morally indistinguishable cases should not be treated differently by law.

Minor premise: Acts of letting die are morally indistinguishable from acts of mercy killing or euthanasia.

Conclusion: Therefore the law should not treat acts of mercy killing or euthanasia differently from acts of letting die.

Whilst the conclusion does follow logically from both premises, we would contend that the premises are seriously flawed and so the conclusion based on them should be rejected.

The minor premise has already been examined above, where we concluded that there are important moral differences between acts of letting die and acts of mercy killing or euthanasia. These differences lie in both intention and in causation of death; in cases of 'letting die' the doctors neither cause nor intend to cause the death of the patient whereas in acts of euthanasia they both intend to cause and do cause the death of the patient. Therefore euthanasia and letting die are not morally indistinguishable and so the minor premise is false.

The major premise, that morally indistinguishable cases should not be treated differently by law, raises issues about the function of law and its relationship to morality. Three essential points should be considered. Firstly, it should be remembered that the function of the law is to safeguard the interests of everyone in the community and not just the interests of a minority, however deserving, against the majority. Secondly, morality is much more complex than the law could ever be. An enforceable, consistent, and comprehensible law is necessarily a relatively 'blunt instrument' compared with the great complexity of moral judgements in particular cases. Yet it is with this blunt instrument that the good of the community must be upheld. So the law has to make distinctions which are unambiguous and comprehensible to ordinary folk, and it cannot possibly follow all the intricacies and nuances of thought and feeling which exist in morality. Thirdly, in treating acts of letting die differently from mercy killing or euthanasia the law is not saying that there is *always* a moral difference between letting die and killing. It is saying only that for legal purposes related to the best outcome for the whole community it is necessary to make this distinction. Indeed, it is not the purpose of law to say which acts are or are not morally indistinguishable.

In addition we would argue that in general there is a significant moral difference between acts of mercy killing and letting die, although it may be possible to produce scenarios where there is no significant moral difference, as shown by James Rachels.[17] It follows from all of these considerations that it is likely that there will be unusual occasions when morally indistinguishable cases will have to be treated differently by law, in the interests of everyone in the community. Although at first sight this situation appears morally undesirable it is not wrong if the good of everyone requires it. Moreover it appears to us that whether it is right or wrong this situation is probably unavoidable.

We have asserted that both premises are false. Nevertheless, if they are accepted by some people the conclusion will logically follow, and so we should consider the consequences of accepting the conclusion. The conclusion suggests that letting die and mercy killing or euthanasia should not be treated differently in law. This would mean treating intentional acts of 'causing death' in the same way as acts of withholding or withdrawing life-prolonging treatment in the context of allowing to die. It would follow then that either both should be prohibited, or both should be permitted.

We have already argued that disastrous consequences for patients would ensue if the withholding or withdrawing of life-prolonging treatment were prohibited. All patients would then be allowed to die only after the application of all possible means to prolong life. Indeed, the phrase 'allowed to die' would no longer have any application; patients would in fact die if but only if they defeated the medical technology! This would have disastrous results; the autonomy of patients and doctors would be grossly infringed by the law, life-prolonging treatments could not be withheld or withdrawn even if their harms outweighed their benefits, thus increasing suffering, and intensive care units would consume the lion's share of the community's resources for health care.

In fact it is much more common to hear it argued that both letting die and mercy killing should be permitted. For example, it might be suggested that withdrawal of feeding from patients in the PVS (persistent vegetative state) is morally indistinguishable from euthanasia and that both should be permitted. The consequences of such a view must be examined.

Proponents of this view would contend that when doctors withdraw feeding from a PVS patient they have intentionally caused the death of the patient because they consider that the patient's quality of life is so poor that he or she should not be kept alive. They would then conclude that if allowing to die is permitted for this reason in the PVS cases then voluntary, and indeed non-voluntary euthanasia for the same reason must also be permitted. This would mean that if it was thought that a person's quality of life was considered so poor that he or she should not be kept alive by means of life-prolonging treatment, then a deliberate act to cause the death of that person should also be permitted. It would then follow that doctors, and indeed perhaps anyone, would be permitted to kill such patients. This would severely weaken the prohibition against killing which currently protects such vulnerable patients. Together with the vast majority of specialist doctors in palliative care in the United Kingdom (according to a survey carried out by the Association for Palliative Medicine in 1997) we consider that any benefit of legalizing eutha-nasia is outweighed by the harms which would result from weakening the prohibition against killing which currently protects them.

5.4 The roles and responsibilities of patients and professionals

The entire WHO statement (see p.4) outlines the duties and responsi-bilities of professionals towards patients in palliative care. In so doing it also describes what patients and their families can expect from health care professionals. The statement is not about any corresponding responsibilities of patients and their families. Nor is it about the responsibilities of society more broadly for providing resources for this care.

Throughout the discussion so far we have stressed the responsibility of health care professionals, especially doctors, to pay attention to the particular patient's problems and to weigh up the possible health benefits of treatments or interventions against their harms and risks when deciding which treatments to offer each patient. We have mentioned the requirement for the competent patient's consent prior to assessments by questionnaire, investigations, treatment, or other interventions such as counselling. In so doing we have described what has emerged as the basic relationship between the professional and patient through the second half of the twentieth century.

In this relationship there exists a balance of powers and responsibilities between patient and professional. The professional is charged with offering investigations and treatments which have a realistic prospect of providing health benefits without undue harm or risk for the patient. This entails using professional knowledge and experience. The corollary of this responsibility is the power to decline to carry out an investigation or treatment which the professional believes will confer no net health benefit and which will therefore probably result only in harm to the patient.

The competent patient has the power to consent to or decline the health care offered. During the last years of the century this *power* has tended to change into a *responsibility* to consent to or decline the care, as the patient's consent has increasingly become a condition which must be satisfied before health care can be given to the competent patient.

During this period patients have not had the power to require professionals to provide a certain aspect of health care, for example a particular investigation or treatment. The professional has retained the power to decline to provide an investigation or treatment, for example where it is excessively harmful or risky in comparison with its foreseen benefit, or where resources (either of manpower or money) are not available to provide it. This power to decline to provide an investigation or treatment is logically necessary if the professional is to be charged with two sets of responsibilities. The first set is the responsibility for offering and providing investigations which are reasonably expected to provide net benefit to the patient as opposed to net harm or risk. The second set is the responsibility for allocation of health care resources, whether in a nationally funded system such as the NHS in the UK, or whether in an insurance funded system where doctors must also use allocate resources honestly within the constraints of the system.

During the beginning of the twenty-first century an important and major change in the patient/professional relationship has been suggested. Some members of the public, some philosophers and some charged with interpreting Human Rights law pertaining to health care have stated that it is patients (and only patients) who should decide which life prolonging measures they should receive, and that doctors ought to be required to provide whatever treatment the patient wishes, whether or not the doctor anticipates that the treatment has any realistic prospect of achieving benefit greater than the harms and risks. Thus the doctor would be required to provide a treatment even if he or she considered that the likely harm and risk far outweighed the benefit sought. We have discussed this issue in Chapter 3 but will review it with particular regard to life-prolonging treatment in this chapter.[†]

In the suggested new model for the professional/patient relationship the doctor must in the end do what the patient asks, either contemporaneously or via an advance statement. Since the doctor lacks the authority to decline, then it should follow that the doctor cannot be held morally or legally responsible for the consequences to the patient, although the doctor's responsibility for the outcome is rarely discussed. Furthermore, the doctor cannot he held morally or legally responsible for the use of resources entailed by the treatment.

The suggested new relationship is advocated by some influential writers. John Harris has argued that a life prolonging treatment must be provided unless the patient consents to its not being provided.[18] Additionally, Jocelyn Downie (as we have seen in Chapter 3), writing in the *Journal of Palliative Care* and with reference to Canadian Law, concludes that 'physicians cannot be allowed or left to determine on their own what treatments should be withheld or withdrawn from competent patients or their surrogates who wish the initiation or continuation of those treatments'.[19] She proposes that if the physician and patient do not agree (as would be the case if the patient requested a treatment which the doctor believed to be overwhelmingly harmful or risky in comparison to its foreseen benefit) then the patient's care should be transferred to that of another doctor who will provide it. If such transfer is not possible, the disagreement must be resolved by a court. These suggestions run so counter to the whole tradition of ethics—not just medical ethics but ethics in general—that it is worthwhile spelling out their implications. We are here repeating some of the arguments of Chapter 3, but the issue is so extraordinary that it is worth repeating.

[†] See footnote, p. 64

The position seems to be that at the beginning of the twenty-first century, at least in wealthy Western cultures, there is a suggestion that the fundamental nature of the professional/patient relationship should change. The suggestion is not that it should change into that of the salesperson or craftsman to customer. For, as we have said, the salesperson or craftsman could and probably should refuse to sell an item which is unfit for the purpose, or carry out shoddy work which would entail risks for the customer. Nor is the relationship like that of other professionals to their clients.

For example, a pet owner could not require a vet to carry out a procedure or treatment to the owner's pet if the vet believed that the requested treatment was harmful to the pet. Neither could a client require a lawyer to carry out a practice improper according to the law nor a parent require a teacher to use a teaching technique which the teacher considered was not in the interests of that particular child. The vet and the teacher carry responsibility for treatment and teaching, and have the authority which must accompany that responsibility.

The suggestion is that the relationship should change into a relationship for which there is currently *no similar or parallel model relationship*. For in this new relationship one party (the professional) is actually required to do to the other party (the patient) that which the professional strongly believes will confer overall harm on the patient. Thus the professional is required knowingly to harm the patient. The problem with this new model relationship is that society has strong moral and legal prohibitions against knowingly harming another. These prohibitions are even stronger where one party is said to have some sort of responsibility or duty of care to the other party. Doctors, nurses, and other professionals are definitely judged to have some sort of duty of care to patients. So it is extraordinary that the proposed new relationship should require them to harm the patient, even at the patient's request. Thus the proposed new relationship runs contrary to the moral rule of not harming others which guides the overwhelming majority of relationships between individuals in society. So the proposed new relationship is morally extremely problematic: it is inconsistent with our fundamental moral principle of not harming others, and with current attributions of responsibility to professionals for the health care they provide.

We should now reflect on what palliative care has to say about the nature of the professional/patient relationship. We have seen that the WHO definition charges professionals with the responsibility for impeccable assessment and treatment of the patient's problems, thus leading us to conclude that the professional must provide only those treatments which will relieve the suffering caused by the symptom or problem, so as to achieve the goal of improving the patient's quality of life. Clearly, if the side-effects are severe, quality of life may not be improved, and if risks are severe life might actually be shortened. Thus, according to the WHO ideology, professionals must be granted the power to decline to provide treatments which would not relieve suffering.

The *OTPM* is helpful in giving insight into the sort of professional/patient relationship which its contributors recommend. Since much of the debate about life prolonging treatment has centred on artificial nutrition and hydration, the section on 'clinical assessment and decision making in cachexia and anorexia' is instructive (Section 8.4.2). The authors, Robin L. Fainsinger and Jose Pereira, avoided reaching a conclusion on the issue of whether or not doctors should be required to provide enteral or parenteral nutrition at the patient's request but where the evidence suggests that there will be no benefit but only harm and risk. They remind us that: 'The common theme of treatment goals is clearly "quality of life". This translates into the goal of relieving nausea, improving appetite and maintaining or gaining weight, and psychological support and education to assist the patient and family in understanding and accepting the benefits and limits of treatment intervention'. They also state that: 'Nutritional support should be viewed as a treatment, subject to the same scrutiny of risk versus benefits as any other treatment'.[20]

Their section reviews the available evidence comprehensively. In their conclusion they note that where patients are in the last few months of their lives 'aggressive treatments and artificial nutrition have been shown, with a few exceptions, to be largely futile and burdensome'. (They go on to recommend that we need to think more, and gather more evidence, about the benefits of such treatments earlier in the illness.) In the context of palliative care, very many patients are in the last few months of their lives. Thus, according to the evidence and the requirement to weigh up the risks and benefits of the nutritional support, one would expect them to conclude that for most patients in the last few months of life artificial nutrition would provide no benefit and would be burdensome, and therefore ought not to be initiated or continued by doctors.

But this is not the conclusion they reach. Instead, they see 'ethical dilemmas' in the decision making process and ask the following questions, without venturing to answer them. 'Does a patient have the right to demand a medically futile treatment (autonomy)?. ... What are the society limitations in determining access to health care and treatment costs (justice)?'

In the next section (Section 8.4.3) of *OTPM*, on 'Dietary and nutritional aspects of palliative medicine', the authors, Isobel Davidson and Rosemary Richardson, similarly review the evidence for benefit from artificial nutrition, but avoid stating an opinion as to whether or not doctors ought to provide such artificial nutrition to patients who ask for it but for whom it is expected to confer no benefit but only the harms and risks of the procedures entailed.[21]

So in terms of the most recent major textbook on palliative care, authors seem to be uncertain about whether a doctor should initiate or continue artificial nutrition where the patient requests it but the evidence suggests it will produce no benefit and will instead impose burdens or risks. At the beginning of the twenty-first century professionals writing on palliative care appear uncertain about what the nature of the professional/patient relationship ought to be. But the nature of this relationship is fundamental to the practice of health care.

We would recommend the following responsibilities in the professional/patient relationship, where the patient is competent or has expressed wishes via an advance statement.

The professional offers to the patient those investigation/treatment options which he/she considers would provide a reasonable balance of benefit to harm and risk in the particular patient's case. There is no objection to, and indeed it might be helpful, if the patient makes suggestions about treatments he/she would want or not want. This process enables joint decision making to commence, and makes the patient integral to the process. But whether or not the patient wishes to take part in this process, he/she must consent to or refuse the investigation/treatment offered.

What the professional cannot do is to force a patient to undergo an investigation or treatment which the adult patient is refusing (even if the relatives want the patient to undergo it). What the patient cannot do is to force the doctor to provide an investigation /treatment which the doctor considers would result in harm and risk exceeding benefit.

Where the patient is incompetent and has not made a valid and relevant advance statement the responsibilities for decision making vary between countries. In the UK at the moment the responsibility for making health care decisions lies with the health care team, unless the patient appointed a lasting power of attorney to make the decision in question. In some other countries, the responsibility to consent to or refuse investigation/treatment on behalf of the patient lies with the relatives. In all cases, the relatives can contribute knowledge of what the patient might have wanted.

5.5 Conclusions

1 The philosophy of palliative care should be consistent with health care ethics in general, and should form an integral part of the latter.
2 The WHO statement that palliative care 'intends neither to hasten nor to prolong death' should be rejected because of its intrinsic ambiguities.
  Health care practitioners may justifiably hasten death as a foreseen but not intended effect of treatment whose aim is the relief of pain and distress at

the end of life, where the benefit of symptom relief outweighs the harm of bringing an inevitable death nearer. Prolonging life is a goal of health care, and is often appropriate in the palliative care context.

3 Guidance for practitioners should state that the benefits, harms and risks of a treatment in the patient's particular circumstances should be weighed up carefully. This includes analysing as far as possible the illness scenarios and ways of dying which are likely to occur with and without the treatments.

4 Professionals bear responsibility for offering competent patients those investigations/treatments which offer a reasonable net benefit. Competent patients bear responsibility for consenting to or refusing to what is offered.

5 In the philosophy of palliative care, and in health care ethics and law generally, 'letting die', in the sense of withholding or withdrawing a life-prolonging treatment when its harms and risks exceed its benefits, must be permitted. Health care practitioners who so act neither cause nor intend to cause the patient's death. The doctrine of double effect is too complex for practitioners to use in clinical practice. It should be replaced by guidance to the effect of points 2–4 above, together with education on the methods of casuistry and using real case scenarios.

6 There is a significant moral difference between intentionally causing the death of a patient by administering lethal medication (mercy-killing or euthanasia) and withholding or withdrawing a life-prolonging treatment because of lack of net benefit with the result that the patient dies of the underlying illness (letting die).

7 The philosophy of palliative care, health care ethics in general, and the law, must continue to uphold the prohibition against killing which protects all members of society. In law, in professional codes and in clinical practice, it is necessary to distinguish between intentional acts which cause the death of patients (acts described as 'killing' or euthanasia) and the withholding or withdrawing of life-prolonging treatment so that the illness causes death (acts regarded as letting die).

References

1 Roy, D. (2004). Euthanasia and witholding treatment. In: *Oxford textbook of palliative medicine*, 3rd edn, ed. D. Doyle, G. Hanks, N. Cherny, *et al.* Oxford University Press, Oxford: pp. 84–97.

2 Roy, D. (2004). Euthanasia and witholding treatment. In: *OTPM* op. cit. pp. 89–93.

3 WHO (2004). *Palliative care: the solid facts.* WHO, Geneva: p. 14.

4 Roy, D. (2004). Euthanasia and witholding treatment. In: *OTPM* op. cit. p. 301.

5 WHO (2004). op. cit. p. 14.

6 WHO (1990). *Cancer pain relief and palliative care.* WHO Technical Report Series 804. WHO, Geneva.

7 **Roy, D.** (2004). Euthanasia and witholding treatment. In: *OTPM* op. cit. p. 85.

8 **BMA** (1999). *Withholding and withdrawing life-prolonging medical treatment.* BMJ Books, London: p. 1.

9 **BMA** (1999). op. cit. p 1.

10 **Roy, D.** (2004). Euthanasia and witholding treatment. In: *OTPM* op. cit. p. 87.

11 **Battin, M. P.** (1994). *The least worst death.* Oxford University Press, New York: pp. 33, 39.

12 **Roy, D.** (2004). Euthanasia and witholding treatment. In: *OTPM* op. cit. p. 84.

13 **Grayling, A. C.** (2005). Right to die. *BMJ*, **330**: 799.

14 **Grayling, A. C.** (2005). op. cit.

15 **Beauchamp, T.L. and Childress, J.F.** (1994). Nonmaleficence. In: *Principles of biomedical ethics*, 4th edn, ed. T. Beauchamp and J. Childress. Oxford University Press, Oxford: pp. 206–11.

16 **Roy, D.** (2004). Euthanasia and witholding treatment. In: *OTPM* op. cit. pp. 89–93.

17 **Rachels, J.** (1975). Active and passive euthanasia. *New England Journal of Medicine*, **292**: 78–80.

18 **Harris, J.** (2003). Consent and end of life decisions. *Journal of Medical Ethics*, **29**: 10–15.

19 **Downie, J.** (2004). Unilateral wihholding and withdrawal of potentially life-sustaining treatment: a violation of dignity under the law of Canada. *Journal of Palliative Care*, **20**(3): 143–9.

20 **Faisinger, R.L., Pereira, J.** (2004). Clinical assessment and decision-making in cachexia and anorexia. In: *OTPM* op. cit. p. 539.

21 **Davidson, I., Richardson**, R. (2004). Dietary and nutritional aspects of palliative medicine. In: *OTPM* op. cit. pp. 546-52.

6

Resuscitation and advance statements

Introduction

Cardio-pulmonary resuscitation (CPR) is a treatment aimed at prolonging life. The immediate aim is to restore the circulation and maintain ventilation. The medium term aim is independence from artificial means of prolonging life such as ventilation so that the patient can leave hospital.

As a life prolonging treatment CPR has practical features which distinguish it from other life prolonging treatments. We will discuss these below, in so far as they are relevant to a discussion on the moral issues which this treatment raises. However, there are two major differences between the decision making process for CPR and the decision making process for other life prolonging treatments. The first is that in the developed world there is an increasing pressure on patients and professionals to make an advance decision regarding CPR in every clinical context except emergency departments. The second is that it is the only treatment for which, in the absence of an advance decision against CPR, it will always be attempted. The assumption is that CPR will be in the patient's best interests, and that the patient would consent.

This practice differs significantly from the process of making best interests judgements for incompetent patients regarding other potentially life-prolonging treatments. It is a treatment about which there is ongoing discussion and controversy, both within the fields of general health care and within specialist palliative care. In the UK, NHS hospitals must have a policy with regard to CPR decision making, and most specialist palliative care units have devised a policy. In contrast, decisions about other life prolonging treatments are not governed by individual policies.

We have included a detailed discussion on decision making in relation to CPR for three reasons. Firstly, since our patients will predictably undergo a cardiorespiratory arrest, a decision on CPR is extremely likely to be needed at some point. Secondly, the decision making process itself is controversial. Thirdly, it seems to be assumed in professional guidance that the decision making process for CPR should differ from that employed for other life prolonging treatments, particularly in respect of presumed consent. Thus it is not surprising that most health care professionals, especially in the context of palliative care, will find themselves reflecting on current practice, and struggling to reach their own conclusions regarding a morally acceptable decision making process, whether they work in generalist or specialist palliative care.

In the following discussion we will examine the existing decision making process recommended by professional bodies, with reference to some of the well known controversies arising from it. We hope that this discussion will clarify the issues and factors which are relevant. We will then propose an alternative decision making process which would be applicable to patients in palliative care and also to those in the acute hospital setting.

The term 'resuscitation' can itself cause confusion, since it is used not only to refer to cardiopulmonary resuscitation but also to measures such as rehydration. In this chapter we are discussing only the process of cardiopulmonary resuscitation, which includes cardiac massage, artificial respiration and the use of drugs and defibrillation as appropriate to restore cardiac rhythm. We are not discussing more general resuscitation measures such as rehydration, methods of maintaining blood pressure etc.

Our discussion will be centred on CPR in the context of palliative care. Currently most patients in whom it is acknowledged that care is now palliative have metastatic malignant disease or progressive non-malignant disease which is anticipated to be fatal and the patient is judged to be in the terminal phase of the illness. Palliative care contrasts with emergency medicine and coronary care units. In the context of emergency medicine the likely balance of benefit to harm and risk is usually less clear, as the underlying diagnosis and prognosis may not be known, or the potential for good recovery may be high, as in instances of near drowning. Similarly, we are not focusing on CPR in the context of coronary care units where potentially reversible arrhythmias may have caused the patient's collapse.

6.1 CPR: a life-prolonging treatment

In the previous chapter we discussed the decision making process for treatments which might prolong life. We concluded that guidance for practitioners should state that the benefits, harms, and risks of a treatment in the patient's particular circumstances should be weighed up carefully. In the context of palliative care this should include analysing as far as possible the illness scenarios and ways of dying which are likely to occur with and without the treatments. We referred to the requirement to justify the provision of a particular treatment, the justification resting upon a reasonable expectation of net benefit.

The BMA, in its guidance on withholding and withdrawing life prolonging treatment (2001), reminds us of this need to justify treatment in the following initial paragraph on the primary goal of medicine:

> The primary goal of medical treatment is to benefit the patient by restoring or maintaining the patient's health as far as possible, maximising benefit and minimising harm. If treatment fails, or ceases, to give a net benefit to the patient (or if the patient has competently refused the treatment) that goal cannot be realised and the justification for providing the treatment is removed. Unless some other justification can be demonstrated, treatment that does not provide net benefit to the patient may, ethically and legally, be withheld or withdrawn and the goal of medicine should shift to the palliation of symptoms.[1]

The BMA makes it explicit that this guidance is intended to apply to CPR as well as other life prolonging treatments.[2] There are two points which should be made about this guidance.

The first pertains to the force of the requirement to justify the provision of a treatment. The BMA has stated that unless there is net benefit the justification for the treatment is removed and concludes that the treatment 'may' then 'ethically and legally' be withheld or withdrawn. We would argue instead that once the justification for providing the treatment is removed then that treatment '*ought* to be withheld or withdrawn' for both ethical and legal reasons. This follows because loss of net benefit means that the harms and risks of the treatment either equal or, more often, are greater than the benefit of the treatment. When this is the case there is surely an obligation, an 'ought', ethically and legally, to withhold or withdraw the treatment. Only in the unusual circumstance that the harms and risks of the treatment are judged to equal the benefit, so that there is neither net benefit nor net harm/risk, is it reasonable to state that the treatment 'may, ethically and legally, be withheld or withdrawn' rather than that the treatment 'ought to be withheld or withdrawn'.

The second point from the BMA guidance pertains to the notion that 'some other justification' could exist and could be demonstrated for the provision of treatment that does not provide net benefit (and so probably provides overall harm and risk) to the patient. This idea that there could be 'some other justification' for providing a non-beneficial treatment, which thus probably confers overall harms and risks, requires analysis in the context of CPR. We shall return to it in the next Section.

Given that CPR is a life prolonging treatment to which the BMA guidance on life-prolonging treatments is intended to apply, it is clear that the judgement of balance of benefit to harm and risk is as necessary in decision making about CPR as it is in decision making about any other life prolonging treatment. Similarly, reasonable expectation of net benefit is required to justify both offering and providing the treatment.

It is somewhat surprising then that in guidance issued specific to CPR, by both the BMA[3] and the GMC,[4] it is recommended that the doctor should carry out CPR if the patient wants it, even when the chances of success are very small or possibly nil. Thus, in the specific guidance the decision in relation to CPR seems to be made on the basis of what the patient wants, rather than on the basis of a positive balance of benefit to harm and risk.

6.2 **CPR compared with other life-prolonging treatments**

Prior to reviewing the arguments for CPR it is important to note that compared with other life-prolonging treatments it has a low rate of success in prolonging life. For a large majority of patients it is ineffective. It could be argued that the criterion for short term effectiveness or success is the achievement of the return of adequate circulation and spontaneous respiration. But in practical terms a more meaningful criterion is the achievement of discharge from hospital. Therefore, this criterion is often used in studies on CPR. Outside of accident and emergency (A&E) departments and coronary care units the achievement of 15 per cent discharge rate following CPR would be regarded as highly successful.

More specifically, the success rate for attempted CPR in cancer patients, and in the context of palliative care for those patients, was reviewed by Kite and Wilkinson. They reviewed the evidence from the available retrospective studies in a comprehensive paper which included reflection on the concept of futility. They concluded that: 'Clinical experience supported by the evidence presented above would suggest that CPR in patients with advanced, progressive cancer who have poor performance status, and irreversible medical problems, can be classified as physiologically futile according to any definition'.[5]

Later, we will make mention of the concept of futility (Section 6.2.3). As Kite and Wilkinson noted, 'a treatment is defined as physiologically futile if it is extremely unlikely to achieve its specified clinical objective'. The objective specified may be short term restoration of circulation and spontaneous respiration, or survival to discharge from hospital. If the patient's condition prior to arrest is taken into account, Kite and Wilkinson noted that: 'survival after CPR is virtually nil for a patient with metastatic disease and poor performance status'.

These clinical circumstances would pertain for the vast majority of inpatients with cancer in a specialist palliative care unit. The extreme lack of effectiveness of CPR in the palliative care patient population, plus its generally poor effectiveness outside that population, should be borne in mind when considering it alongside other life-prolonging treatments.

Nevertheless, as we have noted, professional guidance recommends a decision making process for CPR different from that for other life prolonging treatments. Some significant difference in principle would be required to justify a significantly different process.

We shall argue that CPR as a treatment is not sufficiently different in principle to justify a different decision making process. However, it is important to spell out the arguments both ways because our conclusions regarding the decision making process for CPR, (and the principles underlying it) are vitally important to the discussion. The following three arguments for a different decision making process might be put forward (there may be others).

6.2.1 The 'nothing to lose' argument

In summary, this argument is to the effect that unless CPR is provided and is successful the patient is most certainly dead and is dead immediately.

In the case of other life prolonging treatments such as artificial nutrition and hydration, antibiotics, chemotherapy, the relationship between the disease state, the treatment, and death is nearly always less clear cut. In these examples the patient's life may or may not be prolonged by the treatment, and death, if it does ensue, occurs at some time in the future. In contrast, in the CPR context, where death is inevitable and immediate without successful CPR, people tend to say 'you have got nothing to lose and everything to gain' by attempting CPR. The argument put in more philosophical language is 'the potential chance of prolonging survival, however small, provided it is greater than zero, justifies CPR, since nothing is lost if the attempt is unsuccessful'. In the case of the competent patient one would have to qualify this by adding another condition to the effect that the patient must want CPR. In the case of the incompetent patient, where consent cannot be obtained, one might take the view that provided the chance of success is greater than zero, CPR is in the patient's interests because the alternative to successful CPR is certainly death. Hence, the patient has 'nothing to lose'.

Thus one can see how the argument that the potential chance of prolonged survival, provided it is greater than zero, justifies CPR if the patient wants it, is based on a different underlying principle and a different decision making process from that recommended by ourselves and the BMA in their general guidance on life-prolonging treatments.

In discussing the 'nothing to lose' argument we must recall the decision making process used with regard to other life prolonging treatments. Coronary artery bypass surgery, for example, might prolong life for patients with severe coronary artery disease, but it is not carried out without an assessment of the benefits, risks and harms for the particular patient. Thus a decision might be made not to proceed with such surgery for a patient with associated severe cerebrovascular disease, in whom the risk of CVA during surgery might be considered too high, or for a patient in irreversible renal failure for whom it might be judged that life would be prolonged for too short a time to justify the harms and additional risks of coronary artery surgery. Similarly, where surgery for malignancy is contemplated, a decision is made by the health care team in each case as to whether the harms and risks of surgery outweigh its benefits. Thus when surgery will not be curative, as is often the case in lung cancer, it is not offered to the patient despite the fact that one could argue that it might prolong life.

This process, and the underlying principles, contrasts with the policy of the CPR 'nothing to lose' advocates. There are two main differences. The first lies in the assessment of the consequences of treatment failure. If CPR fails, the patient is usually dead—which he or she would have been anyway had it not been attempted. Hence the argument that there is nothing to lose, as the outcome after failed treatment is not considered worse than the outcome without treatment. But this argument is based on a factually false premise. It is by no means always the case that the patient is not worse off after CPR, as occasionally the patient may survive but with hypoxic brain damage; in which case many would consider that the patient was worse off than being dead. In other words, the patient would have something to lose.

Secondly, and more importantly in terms of the philosophy of palliative care, the 'nothing to lose' argument for CPR is sometimes based on the idea that it does not matter what we inflict upon patients in the time immediately preceding their death, if they are going to be dead shortly anyway. Proponents of this view argue that the failed resuscitation attempt does not harm the patient as the outcome is that he or she is dead. Further consideration of this argument reveals that it is deeply counter-intuitive. We do, in fact, think that it matters what we inflict on people just before they die. Indeed, part of the success and popularity of specialist palliative care rests on the importance placed on the experiences of patients just prior to their death.

In conclusion, the 'nothing to lose' argument does not oblige us to reject for CPR the same decision making processes and underlying principles as are applied to decisions relating to other life-prolonging treatments.

6.2.2 **The 'symbolic value' argument**

In summary, CPR might be said to be an act of attempted rescue, demonstrating the value of individual lives. It might be argued that since a successful attempt at CPR is the only hope of extending survival after cardiorespiratory arrest, and that society has an interest in valuing the life of its members and in demonstrating that valuing, then CPR attempts are justified because they demonstrate that we are prepared to expend human and financial resources on attempts, however unlikely to succeed, to prolong life. There are two problems with this argument.

The first counter argument is that the harms done to those who do not survive the CPR attempt, plus the opportunity costs of the resources expended in the CPR attempts, outweigh the symbolic value benefit of the CPR attempts and the benefits to that very small minority of palliative care patients who might survive. At this point it is important to note that, as a life prolonging intervention routinely attempted, CPR is remarkably unsuccessful, whilst at the same time being invasive and undignified. The expectation of net benefit from other life prolonging treatments such as chemotherapy, surgery, and artificial nutrition and hydration is much higher. Such treatments usually carry a greater than 15 per cent chance of achieving their physiological goal, and frequently with fewer harms and risks than CPR. Thus, in the case of CPR, it is particularly important to weigh up the benefits harms and risks of CPR in the individual patient's case, since the likelihood is for many patients that the treatment will confer no benefit and only harms.

Professional values regarding CPR are likely to be different from community values where those professionals are correctly informed about the benefits, harms, and risks of CPR. This difference in values is likely to cause misunderstandings in relationships between individual doctors and patients and between the profession and the public. The only solution would appear to be deliberate attempts to educate the public about the poor survival rates following CPR in general, and the exceedingly poor results from attempted CPR in palliative care patients. It is interesting that there appears to be almost no interest in such public education campaigns—maybe this is because such a campaign would essentially be conveying 'bad news'.

The second, and more powerful, counterargument is that it is not reasonable to argue that the symbolic benefit to a community of a medical procedure could ever justify providing that procedure to a patient where it was the doctor's clear judgment that there would be no net benefit, and only harm, as a result of the procedure. An individual patient should not be harmed for the sake of a nebulous symbolic community value.

6.2.3 **The 'low cost' argument**

In summary, this argument is to the effect that CPR is always worth a try since it does not consume resources to any significant extent in comparison to other life prolonging treatments.

The resource implications of many life-prolonging treatments, such as ventilation, renal dialysis and chemotherapy are widely understood amongst the public and health care professionals to be significant. In contrast, the perception given by contemporary television dramas is that CPR is a brief intervention which consumes little in the way of human or financial resources and results either in a dead patient or one who is rapidly able to recover and leave hospital. Thus it is likely that there will be a misperception regarding the resources required for CPR. The consequence is that discussions about the moral issues pertaining to CPR rarely consider resource allocation issues because the resource implications are wrongly thought to be insignificant.

The true situation is rather different. The mere provision of CPR which has any chance of being effective requires the continuous presence in an acute hospital of a cardiac arrest team. This group of professionals must all be trained in the procedure. The UK Advanced Life Support course alone requires three whole days of training and must be repeated at regular intervals to maintain skills. A district general hospital with 800 beds in a routine audit recorded an average of about 1.5 cardiac arrest calls each day.[6] At each call the entire team immediately ceases whatever they are doing to rush to the arrest site. This process necessarily disrupts the care of other patients and is costly in terms of staff time.

If the CPR attempt succeeds in restoring the circulation it is very likely that the patient will require ongoing support in a high dependency unit, possibly a coronary care unit or intensive care unit, and may require ventilation.[7] A high dependency unit bed constitutes a very significant resource in terms of skilled manpower, equipment, and money. Moreover, high dependency beds are in relatively short supply in the UK. This means that just processes for allocating the high dependency beds are required. The relevance of this for palliative care is that it will frequently not be considered morally justifiable to give a high dependency unit bed to a patient who is already terminally ill rather than to a patient who has a prospect of longer term survival. The stark reality is that the high dependency unit resource required to maximize the resuscitated patient's chance of survival to leave hospital may not be available because it is already in use by a patient who has a better prospect of survival.

There is therefore a real resource issue in relation to provision of CPR, just as with other life prolonging treatments. The costs of CPR for every patient who survives the initial event and survives until discharge from hospital must be taken into consideration, just as the costs of renal dialysis and ventilation are taken into account when provision is made, on a finite basis, for these other life-prolonging treatments.

In concluding this section we must note here that we are not using an argument sometimes employed by others who argue against the standard provision of CPR—that CPR should not be provided where the clinicians believe it to be 'futile'. We shall not pursue this argument because it is well-known that the term 'futility' is controversial and there is already a large amount of literature on the subject.[8] In terms of the conceptual framework we are recommending that the term 'futility' can simply be by-passed. The important point is that for medical intervention to be justifiable there must be net benefits over harms and risks. It has been our contention that this needs to be shown for CPR as much as for any other treatment. We must now consider the impact of that view on clinical practice. For clarity we have divided the discussion into two sections, pertaining respectively to competent and incompetent patients.

6.3 **CPR decisions and competent patients**

Should competent patients be asked if they want CPR in the context of palliative care? Clearly, patients receiving palliative care are terminally ill. When cardiorespiratory arrest is anticipated as a result of progressive disease and foreseen organ failure, it is essential to question whether patients should be asked whether they would like CPR, granted the overwhelming likelihood of failure and accompanying harms, especially in palliative care.[9]

Nevertheless, it might be argued that the doctor should not unilaterally decide not to provide CPR without first discussing it with the patient. But 'discussing it with the patient' is an ambiguous statement with two possible interpretations. Firstly, it might mean discussing it in a neutral way which implies that CPR is a possible option if the patient wants it, although this line of discussion might leave the clinician in an awkward position. If, after the neutral discussion, the patient decides that they want CPR then the clinician must either provide a treatment which he believes to be harmful, simply because the patient wants it, or deceive the patient by not providing it in the event. Secondly, 'discussion' might mean providing the patient with a sensitive explanation of the reasons why CPR will *not* be attempted. This is surely the preferable course.

But this is not the view of the BMA and the GMC who clearly feel that in these circumstances, where death is foreseen due to advancing and irreversible disease, then the patient should be offered CPR. The GMC states:

> Where a patient is already seriously ill with a foreseeable risk of cardiopulmonary arrest, or a patient is in poor general health and nearing the end of their life, decisions about whether to attempt CPR in particular circumstances ideally should be made in advance as part of the care plan for that patient. A patient's own views, about whether the level of burden or risk outweighs the likely benefits from successful CPR, would be central in deciding whether CPR is attempted. It is important in these cases to offer competent patients [...] an early opportunity to discuss their future care and the circumstances in which CPR should or should not be attempted.[10]

Similarly, the BMA states: 'where competent patients are at foreseeable risk of cardiopulmonary arrest, or have a terminal illness, there should be sensitive exploration of their wishes regarding resuscitation.'[11]

But what does 'sensitive exploration of their wishes' mean in practice? If it turns out that the patient wishes CPR to be attempted, is the professional to say that notwithstanding his or her wishes, it will not be provided? Clearly, no one would endorse such a policy. In other words, 'sensitive exploration' here really means an offer to attempt CPR if the patient wants it. But guidance of this nature is impossible to justify given that there is evidence regarding the notable lack of success of CPR in patients whose death is anticipated from cancer. For example, Ewer *et al.* found that of 171 patients who experienced an anticipated cardiac arrest and underwent CPR, none survived.[12] This concurs with the overview by Dr Kite quoted earlier. The only possible justification for the guidance pertaining to terminally ill patients would be that it is necessarily a benefit to provide any treatment which the patient wants, regardless of the balance of benefit to harm and risk. This issue is discussed in Chapter 3, Sections 3.6–3.8, pp. 62–68 and in Chapter 5, Section 5.4, pp.117–122 with reference to life-prolonging treatment.

It might be argued that patients would decide *not* to accept CPR if they are sensitively informed of its failure rate. However, there is some evidence to the contrary. In a study of patients with metastatic colorectal cancer it was found that when informed, 63 per cent of the patients wanted CPR in the event of a cardiopulmonary arrest.[13]

What should a doctor do if a patient insists on CPR in the face of the relevant evidence of its failure? The professional guidance on this issue is at best confusing and at worst completely internally inconsistent. The GMC states that: '[one] should usually comply with patients' requests to provide CPR, although there is no obligation to provide treatment that you consider futile'.[14]

The BMA states that: 'doctors cannot be required to give treatment contrary to their clinical judgment, but should, whenever possible, respect patients' wishes to receive treatment which carries only a very small chance of success or benefit'.[15]

From these statements one might reasonably deduce that the responsibility for the CPR decision lies mainly with the patient, or perhaps equally with the patient and doctor, but this is not the case. The responsibility actually lies with the doctor in that he or she is accountable for the treatment provided. Only if the patient refuses the CPR treatment offered does the responsibility pass to them. The responsibility for offering and providing the treatment lies with the doctor. Thus the BMA states: 'The overall responsibility for decisions about CPR and DNAR orders rests with the consultant or GP in charge of the patient's care'.[16] Thus one cannot evade responsibility for offering CPR or providing it, nor can one pass the responsibility for so doing to the patient.

The BMA and GMC seem to want the patient's choices to hold great sway in the decision, to the extent that they appear more important than the likely balance of benefit to harm and risk, and yet at the same time the patient bears no responsibility for the CPR attempt. This is not only irrational, it is also potentially very unfair to the doctor who may later be held to account for carrying out a harmful procedure (with no reasonable prospect of benefit) even though they were acting in accordance with professional guidance and the patient's wishes.

Of course, it could be argued that doing what the patient wants is itself a benefit, even if the consequences are not beneficial. This is a deeply counter-intuitive position in most contexts, and certainly in the context of CPR, where the patient's only experience and knowledge base for the want is likely to have come from a medical 'soap opera'. No doubt we are all pleased when we are told that our wish will be granted. But any immediate satisfaction from that knowledge will be vastly outweighed by the bad consequences of an unsuccessful attempt at CPR.

It seems, then, that the guidance of the BMA and the GMC is implying important consequences for the fundamental nature of the doctor patient relationship in society, and possibly for other broader societal values. The case of CPR becomes even more important because it is being used as a basis for changing the nature of the doctor patient relationship, and for changing the nature of decision making within it.

What appears to be happening here is that the doctor is being expected knowingly to harm the patient, and to take responsibility for so doing. This is a major change in the doctor patient relationship, but to what model of relationship does it change?

It does not become a customer-salesperson relationship, for even in this relationship the salesperson may not intentionally and directly harm the customer in anything like the way that an unsuccessful CPR attempt harms a dying patient. This new relationship becomes one for which there is currently no model (see Chapter 3, Sections 3.6—3.8 and Chapter 5, Section 5.4). For it is a relationship where the doctor is required to do whatever the patient competently requests, regardless of the harm which the doctor believes and foresees will follow, and without any benefit. There is no similar relationship which society sanctions.

6.4 CPR decisions and incompetent patients

Decisions made for incompetent patients must be made on the basis of a judgement regarding the patient's best interests. This judgement requires consideration of two factors. The first is the expected balance of benefit to harm and risk of the treatment. The second is what can be known of the patient's wishes. Thus there is a requirement to speak to those who know the patient well, and to take into account any advance statement. The situation is similar to that for competent patients in that the patient's advance request for CPR, or presumed wish to have CPR, is considered in the same way as the competent patient's request for CPR. An additional problem is the inability of the doctor to check what the patient would wish on the basis of correct information about the current clinical circumstances.

Thus for the incompetent patient the same issues arise as those already discussed for the competent patient. The same problems in the nature of the doctor-patient relationship pertain.

6.5 Positive recommendations for CPR decision-making

So far we have argued that CPR ought not to be considered as a treatment to which a different process of decision making should apply. It is not different in morally important ways which might justify a different process. Moreover, the decision making process being advocated by current guidance must fundamentally alter the doctor patient relationship. This latter issue is inadequately considered in the current controversies surrounding CPR. Our view is the one which has been accepted by professional bodies and practising clinicians for a century and more: that whether the patient be competent or incompetent the treatments offered and carried out should be based on a 'best interests' standard, unless of course the competent patient refuses the treatment or the incompetent patient has made an advance statement refusing it. Thus if the treatment clearly does not carry an expectation of net benefit, but instead of only harm or risk, it ought not to be offered or provided, even if the patient wants it.

Recognition of the poor outcomes of CPR generally in the acute hospital setting and increasing awareness of the harms and risks of treatments such as CPR suggest that an alternative approach to the problem is required. We propose the following alternative approach.

In the acute hospital setting, but outside of the A&E and coronary care units, a better standard of care might be provided by removing the focus of decision away from CPR. The idea is that rather than focusing on CPR as a life-prolonging measure, attempts should be made using validated assessments to identify when patients are at risk of an arrest. The assessments are based on simple bedside observations, for example of cognition, respiratory rate, blood pressure and urinary output. These parameters are measured when there is concern that a patient's condition appears to be deteriorating, and following a simple scoring system the patients who are predictably at risk of cardiorespiratory arrest are identified.

Once a patient has been so identified, a decision is made as to which treatments would now be appropriate to attempt to prolong life, and which would not be. In the context of palliative care for a terminally ill patient with a short prognosis and poor performance status it would probably be decided that some treatments were excessively burdensome to the patient in comparison with their potential benefits. The patient may still be competent and may be able to participate in the decision.

For patients with a better prognosis, once the deterioration has been assessed and the risk of arrest identified, then an outreach team from the high dependency unit can asses the patient and institute measures to try to reverse the deterioration, possibly including transfer to the high dependency unit. If those measures fail then clearly the patient's condition is irreversible and at that point a decision not to proceed to CPR is made, on the basis that there is no further potential for significant prolongation of life.

The advantage of this sort of policy, which is applicable only outside the A&E and coronary care environment, is that treatment measures to prevent cardio-respiratory arrest are initiated, hopefully giving a better chance of prolonging life and more time for considered decision making. For patients who are known to be terminally ill and with a poor prognosis a decision is made not to proceed with the more aggressive life-prolonging measures and not to attempt CPR when death occurs. Ideally, when this policy is followed, CPR is not carried out at all, other than in A&E and coronary care units. The energies of personnel such as members of the current resuscitation teams are instead invested in attempts to prolong life, when appropriate, prior to the point of cardiorespiratory arrest. When those attempts fail, CPR is not attempted as it is clear that death is inevitable because attempts to reverse vital organ failure have not succeeded.

Our proposals are not likely to be acceptable to proponents of the notion that patients must receive life-prolonging treatments which they request, regardless of the likelihood of net benefit. But we believe that this sort of policy would yield more overall benefit for patients, and much less harm than many current resuscitation policies, which are fraught with the many problems we have already discussed.

6.6 Advance statements

In the context of palliative care it is clear that treatment decisions, including those pertaining to life-prolonging procedures, will sometimes be required on behalf of patients who no longer have capacity to consent to or refuse treatment offered. At the very end of life metabolic changes leading to confusion or diminished consciousness cause very many patients to have periods of such incapacity.

In recent years it has become accepted practice for competent patients to make known in advance their wishes regarding treatment at a future date when they have lost competence. Such statements may be written, or may be witnessed oral statements. They are often referred to as 'living wills' and were previously called 'advance directives'. Their use in health care has been relatively recent, and the first detailed professional guidance was produced in the UK by the BMA in the early 1990s.[17]

The philosophy of palliative care has traditionally emphasized the importance of respecting and enhancing the patient's autonomy. With regard to patients who it is anticipated are likely to lose that autonomy the question arises as to whether they ought to be encouraged, or even directly asked, to make advance statements and in particular to consent to or refuse treatments in advance. This is seen as a way of continuing to exercise some form of autonomous choice even when actual autonomy has been lost.

We have already noted that with regard to CPR professional guidance recommends that patients be asked to make an advance statement where cardiorespiratory arrest is foreseen. Should this practice be extended to other life-prolonging treatments, such as artificial nutrition and hydration, or to other treatments for symptom relief, such as sedation at the end of life? If we are to ask patients to make advance statements, are we doing so in order that patients will be more likely to receive the treatment they would wish, or in order to make decision making easier for the doctors, or in order to protect doctors against complaints by relatives and potential litigation?

To address these issues we shall first review the arguments in favour of making advance statements, and will reply to each giving the counter arguments.

6.7 Arguments in favour of advance statements

6.7.1 Giving patients what they want

Advance statements may be statements of the patients' values and goals in life, or their requests for certain treatment or refusals of treatment in certain circumstances, or may be statements about their wishes in terms of place of death. An obvious aim and advantage of these statements is to increase the likelihood that the care the patient receives will be that which he or she would wish for.

Currently, with the exception of CPR, patients are not actually asked to made advance statements about treatment as a routine. However, patients may soon be asked to make advance statements regarding their preferred place of care. The WHO guidance of 2004 makes it clear that one of the hallmarks of a good service is whether the patient is able to die in the place of their choice.[18] In order for this standard to be applied patients must clearly be asked to make an advance statement regarding their preferred place of care just prior to death and place of death.

There are particular advantages in making advance statements in the palliative care context rather than when the patient is in good health and has no known serious illness. When the patient is in good health it is not known what the likely future illness scenarios might be, and so it is difficult to express preferences for future treatment since the future clinical circumstances cannot be foreseen.

In contrast, in the palliative care context the nature of the life threatening illness is known and so it is often possible to foresee the likely future scenarios and decisions which may have to be made. For instance, we know that in pelvic tumours ureteric obstruction and renal failure may occur and stent insertion would then be considered. Thus in the palliative care context it is easier for the patient to be informed regarding likely future scenarios and to make advance statements which will actually be applicable in the clinical circumstances which later arise. Moreover, any advance statement the patient makes is more likely to be known to be valid because it will be known that the patient was informed, and not coerced, when the statement was made. This situation contrasts with statements made years earlier by patients then in good health.

So, in the context of palliative care, it can be argued that advance statements are more likely to be valid and applicable to future clinical circumstances than advance statements made when the patient is in good health. Thus in palliative care the statements are likely to result in patients receiving the care they would wish.

6.7.2 Facilitating best interests judgements

Doctors, as part of health care teams, are obliged to make best interests judgments regarding care and treatment for incompetent patients. The two components of these judgments are the balance of benefit over harm and risk of the proposed treatment, and whatever can be known of the patient's wishes. The existence of an advance statement makes clear the wishes which the patient felt it most important to declare prior to losing competence. This clarity does make it easier for professionals to take into account a reliable statement of the patient's wishes. The alternative, of asking family what they think the patient would have wanted, is more difficult for professionals and the information so obtained is less reliable.

6.7.3 Making life easier for the family

It is often difficult for family members, particularly in a distressing situation, to be asked what they think the patient would have wanted in the clinical circumstances which have arisen. Frequently the patient will not have discussed with the family either those clinical circumstances or the particular treatment in question. Yet the family must be asked to try to judge what the patient would have wanted in order to assist the health care team to make the best interests judgment. The presence of an advance statement much reduces the responsibility of the family for judging what the patient would have wanted. Furthermore, if the patient discusses with the family the contents of the advance statement then this process can foster openness about the situation, enabling patient and family to support each other and perhaps draw closer.

6.7.4 Avoiding waste of resources

If there is doubt about the best interests judgment resources are likely to be expended on life prolonging treatment unless it is known that the patient did not want the treatment. Since most advance statements contain elements of refusal of life prolonging treatments they reduce the use of those (unwanted) treatments and so save resources. Those resources can then be used for the benefit of other patients. This can have a major impact on resources in a publicly funded health care system such as the NHS. It is often not appreciated that the cost of a life-prolonging treatment is not simply that of carrying out the procedure, but is also the cost of caring for the patient, who may be very dependent, after the treatment has prolonged life.

These are all reasons to support encouraging patients to make advance statements, verbal or written. But there is a sense in which encouraging patients to make advance statements can verge on compulsion. We have indicated that CPR is the most common example, but artificial nutrition and hydration, stent insertion for obstructive uropathy in renal failure, or antibiotics and assisted ventilation in motor neurone disease are other examples where a line may be crossed from encouraging patients to make advance statements to putting pressure on them to do so, or even forcing them to do so. Despite the advantages listed, there remains the question as to whether it is justifiable even to encourage patients in the palliative care context to make advance statements. The disadvantages of such statements are considered next with reference to the advantages listed above. They serve as counter-arguments to the policy of encouraging or pressuring patients to make them.

6.8 Arguments against advance statements

6.8.1 Difficulties of interpretation and enactment

Statements of values and goals are often so vague as to offer no actual guidance as to what the patient would want in the circumstances. For example, a patient who describes himself as a 'fighter' in an advance statement is not declaring what it is he is fighting for, whether it be life only or whether it be life with independence and mental capacity. Statements of values and goals leave others with the responsibility for working out what the patient would have wanted in the current clinical situation. There is much scope here for error in interpreting from the statement what the patient would have wanted. Worse still, there is scope for disputes between family members or between family and the health care team. The responsibility for interpreting these values or goals statements can lead to family guilt, as they strive to work out what the patient would have wanted, and knowing that their comments will influence the patient's treatment.

Furthermore, advance requests for treatment are not legally binding on health care professionals, so patients will not receive the treatment they request if either it is considered to be clinically inappropriate (i.e. harms and risks clearly exceed expected benefit), or if it cannot be resourced. This latter condition is far more likely to occur in a publicly funded system such as the NHS, where life prolonging treatments such as renal dialysis and certain expensive drug treatments are rationed.

In the UK advance refusals of treatment are legally binding only in restricted circumstances, and it is by no means the case that an advance refusal will ensure that the patient does not receive the treatment. In order to be legally binding two conditions must be met; the statement must be held to be both valid and applicable to the current clinical circumstances. The health care team must take reasonable steps to ensure that the statement was valid, which means that the patient was competent and adequately informed when it was made and was not coerced. The statement should also be dated and witnessed. If there is doubt regarding its validity, it will not be legally binding on doctors. Furthermore, the refusal must be judged to be applicable in the circumstances which have arisen. The statement is applicable if the circumstances which have arisen are those which the patient envisaged and those to which the statement was intended to apply.

It is interesting that the most recent UK law has made it significantly more difficult to formulate an advance refusal of treatment which will be legally binding.[19] It is now, and will be in future, relatively easy for health care professionals to judge that an advance refusal fails either the test of validity or that of applicability. Once it has failed either of the tests the health care professionals can legally proceed with the life prolonging treatment.

Patients making advance refusals of treatment may be seeking the outcome of death as a result of the natural cause of their illness, rather than a prolonged life in deteriorating health. But in some situations refusing the treatment may not result in death but may result in continued life in a confused and dependent condition which the patient may not have wanted. For example, a patient in the palliative care context who has had bisphosphonate treatment once for hypercalcaemia may make an advance statement refusing that treatment again, in the belief that death is likely to result very quickly. But death may not result and the patient may remain in a confused condition and possibly with the additional burden of other symptoms due to the raised calcium.

Thus it is clear that advance statements may not make it easier for patients to receive the treatment they do want and not to receive the treatment they do not want.

6.8.2 Best interests and the duties of doctors

The problems of interpretation of statements pertaining to values and goals have already been described. Assessment of validity and applicability are also extremely difficult, the more so if the statement was not made in partnership with the current health care team. Where statements were made years previously it is frequently not possible to ascertain exactly what information the patient was given or if the patient was put under any pressure. Where applicability is concerned, it is often difficult to know whether the circumstances which have arisen are those to which the patient intended the statement to apply if the clinician was not involved in making the statement, or if the statement is not absolutely specific regarding treatments and circumstances. It is clearly extremely difficult to judge whether a patient's decision regarding treatment whilst still competent is sufficiently at variance with an advance refusal to invalidate that refusal.

These difficulties in interpretation, and assessment of validity and applicability can make it more difficult for clinicians to make best interest judgements in the presence of an advance statement. In the context of the philosophy of palliative care, additional difficulties arise because of the emphasis on quality of life. The goal of palliative care is to 'improve the quality of life of the patient and family'. But following an advance statement, be it requesting treatment or refusing it, may clearly not enhance the quality of life of either the patient or family, thus presenting the clinicians with a moral conflict. In particular, providing (or not providing) treatment according to the patient's wishes may result in a diminished quality of life for the family. Given the philosophy of palliative care, which ascribes equal importance to the welfare of the family and the patient, advance statements can pose almost unresolvable conflicts of aim and principle.

If patients must be asked where they wish to be cared for and to die many will say that they would prefer to die at home. When the time comes, and the patient is confused or has diminished consciousness and thus is incompetent, doctors may recognize that granting the patient's request to die at home may place severe burdens on the family, particularly a single elderly caring spouse, jeopardizing the quality of life and possibly the health of the family. But failing to improve or damaging the quality of life of the family is clearly contrary to the philosophy of palliative care. So the existence of the patient's advance statement, which UK health care teams have now been told they should ask the patient to make, actually makes decision making more difficult morally for specialists in palliative care because of the specialty's stated goals.

Alternatively, patients may state in advance that they wish to be cared for and die in the specialist palliative care unit or 'hospice'. But such specialist palliative care beds are a restricted resource, and in the UK eligibility criteria for specialist palliative care will now have to be met in order to ensure that this restricted resource is given to those patients who need it the most in terms of complex symptom control or other problems.[20] Asking patients where they would like to be cared for and where they would prefer to die is problematic for health care professionals as it implies that the wishes stated will be granted. In fact the necessity for justice in resource allocation and national guidance on that resource allocation will mean that it is not possible to grant the requests of many patients who would wish to be cared for (often for long periods) and later die in specialist palliative care facilities.

The very issue of whether or not to encourage patients to make an advance statement is often problematic for health care professionals. In the context of palliative care patients will clearly require adequate information about the likely future scenarios in order to make such statements and this necessitates giving those patients information about possible future situations, which may be unpleasant and some of which will never arise. It is difficult to judge whether the contemplation of these scenarios will be a net benefit to that patient or whether it will engender anxiety or fear or depression unnecessarily.

Similarly, if a patient who is still competent presents the health care team with an advance statement it is necessary to ensure that the patient still wishes the statement to stand and does not want any modification to it. These questions will need to be asked if there is a significant change in the illness situation in order to check that the patient wants the statement to remain valid.

When health care professionals are presented with advance statements once the patient is incompetent, they may feel morally uncomfortable with either advance refusals or advance requests for treatment. We shall discuss these in turn.

Advance refusals may be perceived as so morally problematic by doctors that they react by attempting to get round them! This reaction is not based on any malicious intent but arises for the following reasons:

1 Reluctance to withhold or withdraw a treatment which they think is in the patient's best interests in terms of the balance of benefit to harm and risk

2 Reluctance to withhold or withdraw a treatment when doing so will possibly result not in death but in survival in a condition which it is considered the patient would not have wanted. The example of the patient refusing treatment for hypercalcaemia applies. Similarly, withholding nutrition and hydration in the immediate period after a cerebrovascular accident may not result in death but may result in weakness which prolongs and makes more difficult the patient's recovery.

3 Judgements regarding what ought to count as 'basic care' rather than life prolonging treatment can be very difficult. Patients cannot decline basic care which includes basic hygiene, the offer of oral food and fluids, and measures deemed essential for the patient's comfort. The problem is the last category. Antibiotics might in some circumstances be considered life-prolonging treatment but they might also be judged the best way of making the patient with a chest infection more comfortable. The available UK professional guidance from the BMA and GMC does not address this problem.

Advance requests for treatment may give rise to the following problems for health care professionals, especially doctors:

1 The requests may be seen as changing the patient-doctor relationship into that of the customer-salesperson. This means that the doctor provides whatever the patient asks for, even if the doctor has grave reservations about the balance of benefit to harm and risk which is likely to result.

2 At the same time the doctors will have a desire to do what the patient wants. These conflicting imperatives cause moral tensions for the doctors who are not able to discuss the issues with the (incompetent) patient.

3 Requests for treatment, if granted, may consume resources and so deprive other patients of more beneficial treatments. This is an issue not just for publicly funded health services like the NHS. Even if the patient is paying for the treatment, either personally or via insurance, the skilled manpower resources such as intensive care unit staff are likely to be in restricted supply, and money is not necessarily able to procure more staff with the necessary skills. It would clearly be unjust to allocate intensive care unit beds on the basis of patients' requests, either contemporaneous or in advance, rather than on the basis of potential net benefit.

4 The moral problems of requests for CPR in the context of palliative care have already been discussed.

6.8.3 Advance statements and family problems

The existence and use of the advance statement may actually make life more difficult and distressing for the patient's family in the following circumstances.

Where family members do not wish to contemplate the future illness and death of the patient, the formulation and existence of the statement forces them to confront the stark reality. Family members, like patients, may sometimes cope better if allowed a measure of denial. The advance statement makes it more difficult for them to cope in this way, and so may diminish the quality of life of some family members.

When the advance statement is being discussed between the patient and family, the family may disagree with the patient's advance requests and refusals and this may be deleterious rather than helpful for their mutual relationship at this crucial time.

Disputes between health care professionals and the family regarding interpretation of the statement may be stressful and very distressing for the family. Conflict may arise in relation to either refusals or requests for treatment or the interpretation of values and goals statements.

Finally, the family in bereavement may feel anger at the (deceased) patient for two reasons: either 'giving up' in the case of advance refusals of treatment, or for requesting life-prolonging treatment, especially where the latter results in prolonged survival of the patient in an incompetent condition and possibly consuming the family resources to fund ongoing care.

6.8.4 Advance statements and resources

Advance statements are unlikely to result in diminished use of health care resources for the following reasons:

1 The time taken to inform patients so that they can make advance statements, and then to review those statements with them over time, will

consume significant resources, mainly in terms of the time of senior doctors. Less experienced staff would not have the knowledge and skills to carry out this complex task with patients.

2 Advance requests for treatment could result in vast expenditure on life prolonging treatments, especially if legal force is given to advance requests for treatment as it is to valid and applicable refusals.

3 Some refusals of treatment will result in patients surviving but with a prolonged recovery period or surviving in a very dependent condition, when treatment would have enhanced recovery.

4 Advance statements will always entail uncertainties about interpretation, validity and applicability. Thus health care professionals are likely to seek legal advice via their employing bodies on a relatively frequent basis. Whilst the statement is formulated at no cost the patient, the costs of legal advice, necessary to ensure they are used within the law and so as to avoid successful litigation by some families, will be borne by the health care service rather than the patient.

6.8.5 Additional problems

There are some practical problems with advance statements which may not be foreseen by either patients or health care professionals.

The first is the issue of where the statement is when it is needed (often at relatively short notice) and the necessity for someone to know that it exists, since when it is needed the patient is unlikely to be able to inform the health care team it exists or of its whereabouts. Moreover, the validity of statements made verbally can be questioned.

In emergency situations there simply may not be time to read the statement, check its validity and make a judgement regarding applicability. For example, if CPR is at issue, then it must be attempted immediately and there is simply no time to deliberate over a page long advance statement which has not previously been studied.

When patients travel away from their own GP and local hospital, who may have a copy of the statement or at least know that it exists, the health care team at their new destination will be unaware of the statement which is also likely to be inaccessible in the short term.

6.9 Advance statements and the philosophy of palliative care

Although we have drawn attention to the problems of writing and interpreting advance statements, we also stress that in the context of palliative care these problems are likely to be less grave. The reason for this is that it is more likely that the health care team will know that an advance statement exists and will have the opportunity to confirm its validity. Moreover, since the progress of the disease is more likely to be foreseeable, it easier to formulate an advance statement which will be applicable in the circumstances which will arise later. Thus is it becomes easier for patients to make their wishes and values known. This will be of benefit to patients, their relatives and to professionals.

6.10 **Conclusions**

1 Current guidance from professional bodies is confused and ambiguous, but seems to recommend carrying out CPR if the patient wants it. This would mean the abandonment of the 'best interests' standard for treatment decisions.
2 CPR in fact, is not different from other treatments in ways which might justify a different decision making process.
3 A better policy involves removing the focus of decision making from CPR and directing attention to the identification of patients at risk of cardiac arrest because they are in the latter stages of an illness known to be terminal.
4 Analysis of the arguments for and arguments against encouraging patients in the palliative care context to make advance statements has clearly resulted in a balance against this policy. This necessarily implies that policies which put pressure on patients or coerce them into making such statements will be difficult to defend when thorough analysis is applied.
5 Rather than having a general policy of encouraging patients to make advance statements, discussion which arises naturally in the context of giving information which patients seek is likely to result in preponderance of the advantages of advance statements rather than the disadvantageous consequences.
6 Attributing legal force to advance requests for treatment is very problematic as has been shown in the discussions on both cardiopulmonary resuscitation and advance statements in general.

References

1 BMA (2001a). *Withholding and withdrawing life-prolonging treatment.* BMJ Books, London: p. 1.
2 BMA (2001a). op. cit. p. 7.
3 BMA (2001b). *Decisions relating to cardiopulmonary resuscitation.* BMA, London: Section 5.2.
4 GMC (2002). *Withholding and withdrawing life-prolonging lreatment: good practice in decision-making.* GMC, London: para 89.
5 Kite, S. and Wilkinson, S. (2002). Beyond futility: to what extent is the concept of futility useful in clinical decision making about CPR? *Lancet Oncology,* 3: 638–42.

6 Schusterbruce, M., Scott, A. (2003). *Audit of CPR attempts* (unpublished). Royal Bournemouth and Christchurch Hospitals Trust.

7 BMA (2001b) op. cit. Section 10.3.

8 Kite, S. and Wilkinson, S. (2002). op. cit.

9 Kite, S. and Wilkinson, S. (2002). op. cit.

10 GMC (2002). op. cit. para 86.

11 BMA (2001b). op. cit. Section 5.1.

12 Ewer, M., Kish, S.K., Martin, C.G. *et al.* (2001). Characteristics of cardiac arrest in cancer patients as a predictor of survival after CPR. *Cancer,* **92**: 1905–12.

13 Haidet P, Hamel, M.B., Davis, R.B. *et al.* (1998). Outcomes, preferences for resuscitation, and physician-patient communication among patients with metastatic colorectal cancer. *American Journal of Medicine,* **105**: 222–8.

14 GMC (2002). op. cit. para 89.

15 BMA (2001b). op. cit. Section 5.2.

16 BMA (2001b). op. cit. Section 11.

17 BMA (1993). *Medical ethics today.* BMJ Books, London: pp. 161–4.

18 WHO (2004). *Palliative care: the solid facts.* WHO, Geneva: p. 17.

19 *Mental Capacity Act UK, 2005.* HMSO.

20 NICE (2004). *Improving supportive and palliative care for adults with cancer.* NICE, London.

7

Assessment and treatment of psychosocial and spiritual problems

Introduction

The WHO definition which summarizes the philosophy of palliative care clearly states that practitioners should treat emotional, psychosocial, and spiritual distress: 'Palliative care is an approach that improves the quality of life of patients and their families.... through the prevention and relief of suffering.... by means of early identification and impeccable assessment and treatment of pain and other problems, physical, psychosocial, and spiritual'.[1]

The definition assumes that assessment and treatment of such problems is possible, and then goes on to state that practitioners have a professional responsibility to undertake the task. We shall discuss these assumptions under two headings: firstly, is it the responsibility of health care professionals to undertake this task? (Section 7.1); and secondly, if as we shall suggest, it is neither possible nor desirable for them to attempt to treat such problems, is there an alternative way of approaching them? (Section 7.2). We have discussed the issue of spiritual care in Chapter 2 pp. 33–35, since it is often seen as a domain of quality of life. Nevertheless we shall touch on it again in this chapter.

7.1 Psychosocial and spiritual problems as a health care responsibility

In health care ethics in general there is little emphasis on professional responsibility for psychosocial care in the hospital sector, although recognition of the patient's emotional state has always been considered important in primary care. However, such recognition is different from assuming responsibility for altering the patient's psychosocial and spiritual state, as is suggested by the definition of palliative care.

Since the beginning of the modern specialist palliative care movement there has been emphasis on the importance of enhancing the patient's emotional, social, and spiritual well-being. The concept of 'total pain' emerged early in the history of specialist palliative care.[2] One consequence of this concept was that psychosocial and spiritual care became essential components of pain control, in a situation where pain control was indisputably mandatory. Thus from this time on psychosocial care became an inescapable responsibility for specialists in palliative care.

The term 'total pain' can simply mean the physical pain which the patient perceives, but which we know is influenced by emotional and mental factors via a very complex neurological network. Alternatively, it may be interpreted as including the patient's entire experience of distress resulting from terminal illness. There seems no problem about the first interpretation of 'total pain'— perceived pain has a complex aetiology, in that the final perception of a stimulus has been modified by other factors in the physical and emotional environment of the individual.[3] But there are problems about the second interpretation—which suggests that a clinician should try to alter the patient's psychosocial and spiritual state in order to modify the pain. These problems are the ones which will concern us in this chapter.

The ideal that health care professionals should make it their responsibility to assess and treat patients' psychosocial and spiritual problems, either for their own sake or in order to treat pain, continues today. For example, in the section on emotional issues in the *OTPM* Mary Vachon states that:

> The assessment and treatment of the psychosocial distress associated with terminal illness involve distinguishing between the normal symptoms of adjustment to a terminal illness and the symptoms of a major psychiatric disorder. The skilled practitioner must be able to identify, assess, and, when possible, treat the physical symptoms of the disease together with the increasing debility and changes in social roles and social isolation associated with the disease and the dying process.[4]

The idea that professionals can provide a 'treatment' for a change in social role, or for social isolation, so as to enable the patient to achieve his maximum potential in all respects, is probably unrealistic. It is also very questionable whether the process of normal adjustment to terminal illness produces 'symptoms' which should be 'treated'. We would argue here that assessing and 'treating' the consequences of a normal adjustment process at the end of life amounts to medicalizing an inescapable part of every human life.

The corollary to the ideal of psychosocial and spiritual care is that professionals have in some way failed to discharge their professional responsibility if they have not assessed and treated aspects of the patient's psychosocial experience. It is important to ask whether the roles and responsibilities for both patient and professional are appropriate.

7.1.1 **The patient-professional relationship**

Given that the professionals are supposed to be able to enable the patient to reach out to his hopes and to end his life meaningfully, it is important that the nature of the patient-professional relationship required to do this is fully appreciated. Dame Cicely Saunders does state that this can be achieved *if* the patient is recognized as the unique person he is and is helped with his family and other relationships.[5] This entails a relationship of a close personal nature between professional and patient, for the combination of recognizing the patient's uniqueness and becoming involved in the way he conducts his closest relationships must logically require a close personal relationship.

The reasons for this conclusion are as follows. Becoming involved in the way a person conducts his relationships may entail making some critical comment (albeit constructive) as well as approbation, and only close personal relationships can stand the degree of honesty which serves as a marker of intimacy. Moreover, recognizing the patient's uniqueness in the context of his terminal illness and life will entail feelings of sympathy and compassion which tend to connect the professional to the patient in a personal link. Dame Cicely Saunders seems to be advocating a very genuine and personal concern for the patient. She states clearly that the patient as a unique individual *must matter* to the professional.[6]

One might object that perhaps she means that the patient must matter to the professional simply because he or she is a *patient*, and it is a feature of the traditional professional/patient relationship that every patient's welfare must matter, or be important to, the professional. This sense of 'matter to' does not entail a close personal relationship. However, the stress put by Dame Cicely on the patient's uniqueness, the idea of helping the patient in his/her relationships, and the professional responsibility she describes for enabling the patient to attain the life and death most meaningful *to him* all imply a close personal relationship, not the traditional professional doctor-patient relationship. The latter would seem to have no prospect of achieving the goals that she (and many others in specialist palliative care) set for practitioners.

Other writers outside the field of specialist palliative care are also beginning to advocate a more personal relationship with the patient. This may be because of the development, particularly in nursing, of 'an ethic of caring' which seems to entail a more personal relationship. Anne Scott, a professor of nursing, writes:

> Health care professionals have a duty to engage actively at a level which allows them to gain sufficient insight into the personal world of the patient to perceive the likely implications of certain treatment decisions for *this* particular patient. Engagement of this sort, I suggest, only comes through activating moral imagination. [...] Without

to some extent entering imaginatively into the world of the 'person-who-is-the-patient', it is impossible to achieve much of the understanding upon which compassion depends.[7]

In declaring that professionals have a *duty* to try to gain insight into the patient's *personal world*, Anne Scott is clearly advocating that they try to establish a personal relationship with the patient, for surely such insight could not come from any less intimate relationship. She grounds this duty in the idea that without such insight professionals cannot have compassion, and compassion is seen as central to an ethic of caring in nursing.

This idea is expressed by other writers in the field of nursing. Verena Tschudin, writing on ethics in nursing, gives a description of caring, which is considered to comprise compassion, competence, confidence, conscience, and commitment.[8] The importance of compassion is particularly stressed. Churchill goes so far as to say that in nursing 'Compassion is the groundwork, competence the superstructure'.[9] Thus compassion seems to be a foundation of caring.

In turn, compassion has been described as follows by Nouwen:

> Compassion asks us to go where it hurts, to enter into places of pain, to share in brokenness, fear, confusion and anguish. Compassion challenges us to cry out with those in misery, mourn with those who are lonely, to weep with those in tears. Compassion requires us to be weak with the weak, vulnerable with the vulnerable, powerless with the powerless. Compassion means full immersion in the condition of being human.[10]

At times in Tschudin's discussion the importance of the caring relationship is seen to override other professional issues. For example, she states that:

> The carer is in relation with the care-receiver. That is what care is all about. [...] Anyone who has been at the receiving end of care will say that what matters most is how human the nurse or doctor - or any carer - is. Not how clever, how efficient, how good with the best equipment; no - but how able the carer is to receive the cared-for: that is what matters.[11]

Most patients on the receiving end of care would profoundly disagree with this statement. The technical skill of the surgeon is more important to most patients than his caring relationship with them. The results of a qualitative study on communication by surgeons and oncologists with breast cancer patients showed that: 'the dominant concern was the need to trust the doctors' expertise [...] Expertise was communicated by being a doctor, and by being efficient, acclaimed, or frank'.[12] And the performance of basic but essential nursing tasks to ease discomfort and prevent long hospital stays is surely more important than 'how human' the nurses are. In our view competence in professional skills and knowledge should be regarded as essential—

neither an attitude of caring and compassion nor the establishment of a particular relationship with the patient will achieve the goals of health care, even in the context of incurable and fatal illness. Nor is it clear that the professional has any *right* to thrust such a relationship on a reluctant patient. Harassment by questioning in the name of compassion has little acceptability.

Yet in the specific context of palliative care other writers stress the importance of the close relationship between professional and patient. Mary Vachon, writing on the topic of the stress of professional caregivers in the *OTPM*, notes the following in a section on the manifestations of job stress:

> Peabody stated "the secret of the care of the patient is in caring for the patient". Palliative care encourages such caring and resulting closeness to the patient. Some of the difficulties associated with the care of dying persons may in part be due to the close connections palliative care staff often develop with their patients. Whereas, traditionally, professionals have been taught to maintain a boundary between themselves and their clients, in palliative care very close relationships can and do develop..... Empathic communication demands good listening and may result in the palliative care worker going "beyond the dimensions of listening to emotional realms that are neither easy nor comfortable". The closeness and exposure to repeated difficult illness experiences and deaths may lead to the experience of "Secondary Traumatic Stress" (STS) or compassion stress.[13]

Vachon accepts that the establishment of a close personal relationship is appropriate in palliative care, has acknowledged the likely consequences for the health care professionals, and notes the potential for multiple griefs and losses. But clearly, professionals will suffer this personal grief and loss only if they have established with their patients the sort of close and caring relationship advocated by Scott and Tschudin, and acknowledged by Vachon to be the accepted appropriate relationship between professional and patient in palliative care. We would question whether the attrition on health care professionals consequent upon this close relationship is justifiable. The justification would have to be based on considerable benefits to patients and their families resulting from a close relationship as such. The evidence for benefits of psychosocial care is mentioned later.

It should be noted that the concepts of care, compassion, commitment, and sympathy, which have been 'borrowed' for use in health care ethics, have their origins and a long history in personal relationships which pre-dates their mention in health care. As Christopher Cherry notes: 'they remain embedded in a realm of morals, and ultimately of ethics, which tends towards the personal as opposed to the impersonal, the individual as opposed to the collective, the partial as opposed to the impartial, and the unmanaged as opposed to the managed'.[14]

Clearly, in a managed system of health care such as the UK's NHS, there must be impartiality and concern for the collective good, especially in the face of scarce resources. Christopher Cherry concludes that it is inconceivable and impossible for 'the partial and particular and personal to co-exist with and soften the impartial and the impersonal'. He is clear that the concepts of care and compassion, having their roots and meaning in personal relationships, cannot simply be transposed into a managed system of health care and into the patient/professional role.

We shall later cast some doubt on that view. We have already suggested, and will later develop the suggestion (Chapter 9, Section 9.2.2, pp.203–205) that it is possible for both to co-exist, at least to a limited extent. The interesting point for present purposes however is that 'caring', 'compassion', 'empathy', and like terms have been transformed as they enter a managed care system. Using the terminology we have introduced, we can say that Asklepian notions of special attention to the individual are being professionalized in terms of the concepts of Hippocratic medicine. So we find 'scales' to 'measure' the practitioner's empathy, and incredibly 'tools' to 'measure' the patient's spiritual needs.[15] In other words, the simultaneous desires to retain concepts which are appropriate for personal relationships and also to demonstrate that the practitioners are fully professional leads the professionals to bombard very sick patients with questionnaires and assessments, and put numbers to them. This leads to suggestions (as in the *OTPM* chapter on communication) that in order to assist professionals to detect psychological morbidity 'screening patients with validated questionnaires prior to seeing the doctor might improve detection rates'.[16]

7.1.2 Effect of the recommended relationship on the patient

At first sight, if the establishment of this close relationship solves the patient's psychological, social, and spiritual problems then it would appear to be a good thing for the patient. It must confer some sort of overall benefit on the patient. But we must look at the process of building this relationship, not just at the outcome which it is claimed to achieve.

As mentioned above, a close relationship requires considerable knowledge of the patient. In the first edition of the *OTPM* Mary Vachon suggests two ways 'of approaching an assessment of what causes most concern in a terminally ill person'. She asserts that the first approach involves inquiring into the following; health and well-being of every kind, family and marital attitudes, housing and money worries, sexual and social activities, job and daily life, self-image, and existential issues about illness, invalidism, and death. The alternative approach which she advocates is 'assessing what patients want' and she states that this includes possibilities such as relief of symptoms, better support, firmer security, sustained relationships—both personal and professional, and stronger morale to face the future. She goes on to suggest a number of questions which might entice patients 'who do not want to speak about personal matters' to discuss the areas she is interested in. She adds that: 'Using these approaches the interviewer can begin to assess the areas in which patients will be able to use practical assistance to help them cope more effectively. This will also allow the clinician to decide in which areas he or she is comfortable to intervene and which will require some outside assistance'.[17]

Vachon's description of the recommended professional approach to a patient in the context of palliative care is not unusual. It should be noted that this approach entails a number of assumptions. It assumes that the patient wants some intervention into his or her psychological, emotional, social, and spiritual state, or it assumes that the process of intervention is justified by the benefit to the patient, and perhaps most importantly it assumes (without any evidence) that the patient *consents* to this type of questioning or to any intervention. Where patients are unwilling to divulge the information she seeks, Vachon actually suggests the questions which might cause them to reveal it!

Thus the establishment of this close relationship may not be a good thing for the patient—the latter may be exposed to intrusive or manipulative questioning without consent, and worse still, may perceive that he or she receives essential symptom control and treatment only if he or she acquiesces to such questioning and provides the answers.

In health care generally it is now widely accepted that treatment is not given to competent patients without their informed consent, and that any form of duress or coercion in the process of obtaining such consent is unacceptable. Yet consent in the context of psychosocial care in palliative care is hardly ever explicitly sought. It is the terminal illness of the patient which has caused the patient to seek help, so it is this illness for which the patient has given implied consent for health care. The scope of implied consent is difficult to define, but it suffices to say that we cannot assume that a patient implicitly consents to whatever care interventions the professionals consider would be beneficial. Someone asking for pain control does not necessarily want to explore feelings related to the diagnosis, let alone those related to previous life crises, close relationships, or sexuality. It is certainly disrespectful of patients to embark on personal discussions unless they have indicated a desire or at least willingness to do so.

Of course patients may want help with social, psychological, or spiritual problems, especially once physical distress has been alleviated. It is obviously appropriate to ask frequently what problems the patient wants to address. But there is a subtle and morally important distinction between encouraging patients to talk about their present concerns and asking searching questions which it is difficult to avoid answering. In the context of specialist palliative care patients are often placed in situations from which it is difficult to escape without making personal revelations. It is not morally acceptable to assume that patients want and consent to care for emotional, social, and spiritual distress, and on the basis of this assumption to instigate deeply personal assessments and interventions.

This is a difficult area in palliative care, where professionals (influenced by writings such as those quoted above) are so strongly motivated towards relief of all distress that they tend to assume that the patient, in consenting to give a history of the illness and in permitting physical care and examination, is also consenting to give a personal life history and is permitting the detailed assessment of psychosocial problems that is generally recommended in texts on palliative care. However, the belief that the relief of psychosocial distress is a morally good aim, and a great benefit to the patient, cannot justify attempting to 'treat' these problems without the patient's consent.

The situation in palliative care is confounded by the dependence of the patient on the team for physical care and symptom control. The assumption of consent to psychosocial assessment and intervention leads to the infliction of 'care' on the patient who may find it difficult to refuse this care or even to escape from it, especially if it is 'sold' to the patient in a package in which it is inextricably mixed with physical care and treatment which *is* wanted. It is clearly not morally justifiable to bind different aspects of care together in this way so that it is difficult for patients to select those which they want and to refuse those which they do not want. Yet in the drive for 'holistic' care specialists in palliative care have become almost unaware that they are binding symptom control and physical care together with psychosocial care.

In the context of treating physical symptoms, professionals working in palliative care strive to avoid investigations and treatments which entail invasive procedures or which are associated with harms and risks where the benefits are not large enough to justify those harms. For example, writers describing the assessment of delirium in terminally ill and dying patients in the *OTPM* state that 'Most palliative care clinicians would undertake diagnostic studies only when a clinically suspected aetiology can be identified easily, with minimal use of invasive procedures, and treated effectively with simple interventions that carry minimal burden or risk of causing further distress'.[18]

One must ask whether the investigation of the patient's psychosocial and spiritual condition is a 'minimally invasive' procedure. One must also ask whether any interventions carry only a 'minimal burden or risk of causing further distress'. (We will mention later the additional question of whether psychological, social and spiritual problems can be 'treated effectively'.)

Professionals working in palliative care are exhorted to elicit as many of the patient's 'concerns' as possible. Maguire and Pitceathly writing in the *OTPM* comment that 'If patients fail to disclose their main concerns, attempts to counsel them will be less effective [...] The low disclosure and identification of patients' and carers' concerns may explain, in part, why the prevalence of affective disorders remains high'.[19] The authors go on to state that 'It is crucial, therefore, to understand the barriers to disclosure, learn how to overcome them, and recognize when patients are suffering from depression and/or anxiety'. One must question here whether the aim of identifying depression or anxiety justifies what sounds like manipulative attempts to cause the patient to disclose that which the patient is reluctant to disclose, or would choose not to disclose. In the detail of the text of this section of the *OTPM* the authors do point out that 'negotiation' is important to 'allow patients who find it too distressing to discuss such issues to decline to do so'. Our anxiety is that the overwhelming drive, which the palliative care approach encourages, to seek out information on the patient's psychosocial and spiritual concerns, may encourage intrusive and manipulative questioning. Worse still, it might cause professionals to consider that patients must somehow be forced to divulge deeply personal feelings.

The possibility of medical intervention becoming a source of suffering was recognized by Cassel as follows: 'The failure to understand the nature of suffering can result in intervention which though technically adequate not only fails to relieve suffering but becomes a source of suffering itself'.[20] We would wish to stress that there is a risk that any intervention designed to relieve suffering, even one designed to alleviate psychosocial or spiritual suffering, can in fact become a source of suffering itself. We suggest that some or all of five different types of harm to the patient may result from psychosocial interventions.

Firstly, as we have already said, intrusive and potentially exhausting questioning in the name of assessment of psychosocial and spiritual needs may clearly be a *harm* to some patients. Secondly, a harm may be caused if professionals imply to patients that they have 'un-met needs' in situations where those patients had not recognized any such need. Needs can be identified only by the patient, and not by professionals. There is a danger that professionals assume some unmet needs on the basis of their own experiences, values and beliefs, or on the basis of what they have been taught that patients need. They may then consider it necessary to explore in detail those perceived or assumed needs which the patient may hitherto be unaware of (and therefore not distressed by) or which the patient may not wish to discuss. For example, a nurse may suggest to a patient that she has an unmet need for continuing sexual contact. The patient, whose libido is reduced by hormone therapy and by her illness, may not perceive this need but may be very suggestible and may also think that as a normal woman she 'ought' to have this need. In fact it may be very difficult for her to have satisfactory sexual contact for many reasons. Thus an iatrogenic unmet need may be generated and give rise to distress.

Thirdly, the patient may be harmed if the professional concludes, rightly or wrongly, that the patient's response to circumstances derives from some deep-seated 'hang-up' or unfinished emotional business which the professional thinks the patient 'needs' to sort out. In fact the patient may be too exhausted or simply unwilling to confront a long-term 'hang-up' which was not dealt with even in health. Specialists in palliative care often consider that their role is to help patients to achieve a peaceful and meaningful death. To this end they believe that patients should be encouraged and 'helped' to resolve some issues (often in relationships) that have troubled them for many years in life. As a result of this belief there is a definite risk that the patient may be distressed by being encouraged or persuaded to confront a traumatic issue or relationship.

Fourthly, denial of the diagnosis or prognosis by the patient may be perceived by carers as a need to break down that denial in order to enable the patient to make more realistic life plans and move on towards acceptance of death. But since denial is known to be a protective mechanism, and thus a coping mechanism, there is a significant risk that the patient may be harmed if it is broken down. In our view this risk is justifiable only if the denial is causing the patient to refuse highly beneficial treatment or if the denial itself is causing emotional distress. Even Peter Maguire writes of the dangers of breaking down the patient's fragile defences when he states that: 'Patients use denial as a defence when the truth is too painful to bear. So it should not be challenged unless it has created serious problems for the patient or relative'.[21]

Fifthly, there is a serious risk that the patient's condition may deteriorate while the issues are unresolved and the patient is in a transitional state of even greater distress, confusion, or anxiety. A traumatic death amidst re-awakened and re-lived distress may result. This outcome is clearly a significant harm.

Some of these five harms, or types of iatrogenic suffering, are likely to result from intrusive psychosocial or spiritual interventions. Indeed, they are quite alien to the Asklepian spirit of palliative care. As John Hinton remarks, 'peaceful acceptance has remained the seldom questioned common aim' of professionals in palliative care.[22] Our point is that 'peaceful acceptance' is not encouraged by intrusive and unwanted probing into the patient's private world.

Another line of argument for breaking down the patient's denial used by writers in the *OTPM* is that a benefit to the patient's family may result. For example, Vachon writes that: 'Patients who are single parents with dependent children, or others whose failure to acknowledge their prognosis may jeopardize their family's future may require a somewhat more directive approach'.[23] Our anxiety is that this 'directive approach', adopted for the benefit of the family, may be associated with harm to the patient by destroying his defensive stance of denial. To put the issue more starkly, a vulnerable patient is being used as a means to further the welfare of third parties. We have discussed this moral problem in Chapter 4.

Sometimes it is suggested that distress which the patient is experiencing as a result of family relationships can be relieved by getting the family together in a situation of 'family therapy'. If such therapy is not conducted by someone highly skilled and experienced there is a great risk of harm to all concerned. Even case conferences about the patient's future care can give rise to expression of strong emotions and suppressed family strife may come to the surface. When this happens it can be destructive to all concerned. In the context of palliative care there may simply not be sufficient time and energy from the patient and family to resolve relationship difficulties, so that encouraging people to air their differences may result only in distress.

Leaving aside the considerable risks of harming the patient by psychosocial intervention our view is that sadness, anxiety and a sense of loss in a terminal illness do not constitute or represent any sort of unmet need or problem which should be 'treated'. Rather they are simply natural and appropriate human responses. If this is the case then it is doubtful that the patient would benefit from their abolition, even if that were wanted and possible. It makes little sense to say that sadness, loss, and realistic anxiety are 'needs' which should be met, or that they are inappropriate responses which should be manipulated in some way into alternative responses that professionals believe are more beneficial. In this respect we are in total agreement with the comments made by the WHO: 'Anxiety and depression are normal responses to loss and the threat of loss in lifelong relationships'.[24]

On the other hand we disagree with the *OTPM* section on psychiatric symptoms in palliative medicine where the authors note that: 'Managing psychiatric complications (such as anxiety, delirium, depression, suicide, and desire for hastened death) and difficult psychosocial issues (such as bereavement, loss, family dysfunction) facing patients with terminal illness and their families, however, can test the limits of even the most skilled and experienced palliative medicine practitioner'.[25] The authors are here lumping together two different types of problems—the psychiatric and the normal human experience. The clear implication is that the normal life experiences of 'bereavement, loss, family dysfunction' and perhaps also rational anxiety or rational desire for hastened death, are all states which the palliative medicine practitioner ought to be trying to identify and then 'manage' in some way so as to change them into responses which the practitioner considers to be more beneficial to the patient. This is simply old-fashioned medical paternalism in a new guise!

On the other hand, conditions such as depression, which is common, can and should be recognized and treated. The diagnosis and management of depression is fully discussed in the chapter on psychiatric disorders in the OTPM.[26] Furthermore, anxiety and guilt based on misunderstandings about the aetiology of the illness or about its future progression should be assuaged by giving accurate information and truthful (but not false) reassurance. The WHO repeatedly stresses the importance of giving information, but with regard to anxiety and depression they comment that 'Health professionals who meet people at the very end of these relationships may not be able to influence these basic responses'.[27]

In summary one might say that professionals must distinguish between conditions such as clinical depression or pathological anxiety which are treatable conditions, and normal adjustment responses which include sadness. The latter require no professional interventions, but see Section 7.2 below for our suggestions as to more appropriate professional responses.

7.1.3 The effect of the recommended relationship on the professional

Whilst professionals may gain a great deal from rewarding close relationships with their patients, especially in terms of job satisfaction and enjoyable and stimulating human contact, there are clearly associated harms for them as well as for patients.

The most obvious is the emotional trauma resulting from repeated losses of patients to whom they have become personally attached. Doctors and nurses are able to maintain emotional well-being in specialist palliative care partly because they do not become personally attached to the vast majority of their patients. This is not to say that the patients do not matter to them, nor that they fail to recognize that each person is unique. Rather, it is to say that they matter because they are patients and only as patients—the relationship

remains in the realm of the traditional doctor-patient or nurse-patient relationship, rather than becoming a bond of personal attachment. The formation
of relationships with patients which are close and personal enough to solve the
patient's psychosocial problems, or 'meet the patient's psychosocial needs', is
likely to result in repeated grief and bereavement experiences for professionals.
Such frequent and repeated losses would be unsustainable.

Furthermore, there is a great emotional cost in 'suffering with' the patient to
the extent recommended by those who subscribe to the descriptions of
compassion quoted above. Emotional distress and exhaustion are likely to
result. Anne Scott disputes this and claims that the more the professional
focuses on and becomes imaginatively involved in the patient's circumstances
the less the professional will focus on his or her own distress. She claims that
such a 'patient-directed' practice will allow an enriching and enlarging of the
practitioner's perspectives.[28] But this claim does not take into account the
exhausting nature of trying to absorb and understand the distress of another.
However much one is concentrating on the patient's distress, this does not
decrease the personal impact of witnessing at close quarters the pain and
suffering of others. Indeed, concentrating only on the patient may simply
submerge the practitioner's distress so that it goes unrecognized until it
manifests itself later in mental or physical exhaustion or illness. These latter
outcomes are listed by Vachon in her description of 'Burnout' in professionals
working in palliative care.[29]

Professionals are also likely to suffer feelings of guilt and failure if a patient's
psychosocial distress is not relieved. The assumption that the role and responsibility of the professional is to enable the patient to attain a meaningful death
will inevitably lead to feelings of failure and guilt if patients die apparently still
emotionally or spiritually distressed or with continuing strife in relationships.
Vachon notes the finding that 'Nurses have difficulty with grief if they have not
been able to help the patient die a good death for whatever reason'.[30] Since it is
easier to relieve physical symptoms such as pain than to enable patients to
achieve a meaningful death, much more stress and even depression and guilt
are likely to result from perceived failure to achieve the goals of psychosocial
and spiritual care.

Finally, there is a real possibility that in immersing themselves in their
patient's lives and problems, and in forming close relationships with them,
health care professionals cease to develop their own lives and talents, especially
those outside the work environment. They may increasingly try to meet their
own emotional needs at work. The tendency to do this is aggravated by
spending long hours at work and little at home. However, the main reason
is the emphasis which the philosophy of palliative care puts on responsibility

for the patient's psychosocial well-being which entails close involvement with the patient, in order to assist patients towards an 'ideal' death.

7.1.4 Benefits versus harms of the relationship

One must conclude that there are significant harms for both patients and professionals in forming this close personal relationship. This conclusion is supported by the genuine and pervasive uncertainty, and perhaps controversy, regarding whether the 'interventions' of psychosocial and spiritual care are actually effective. On one hand it is stated in the *OTPM*, in relation to communication and anxiety and depression, that 'Palliation should include treatment and amelioration of all symptoms including psychological ones. There is increasing evidence from well-conducted trials that psychosocial interventions are effective with adult cancer patients'.[31] This statement is based on the results of a meta analysis of randomized studies. In contrast, in the section on psychiatric symptoms in palliative medicine, after interventions for despair, hopelessness, demoralization, and loss of meaning have been discussed, it is noted that: 'Because depression and hopelessness are not identical constructs (although highly correlated) clinical interventions, such as those described above, developed to more specifically address hopelessness and related constructs such as dignity, loss of meaning, demoralization, and spiritual suffering or distress will be important to empirically test and utilize in palliative care practice *if* they prove effective' [our italics].[32] This sentence implies that we do not yet know if these interventions are effective (in contrast to pharmacological and some non-pharmacological treatment of depression). The authors make it clear that research is continuing into the effectiveness of interventions to maintain dignity and to help patients find meaning, peace and purpose in their lives.

A summary of the current situation is given by the WHO writing on psychological interventions: 'A wide range of psychological interventions has been tested in over 150 randomized trials over 40 years. The results were mixed and tended to vary by site of disease and follow-up period, with positive outcomes not being sustained over time'.[33] Thus our first point is that intrusive questioning to identify the patient's psychosocial and spiritual concerns so that an 'intervention' can be applied, is very difficult to justify unless there is strong evidence that the 'intervention' is actually effective. Such evidence does not seem to exist.

Discussion is further hampered by some vagueness as to what counts as an 'intervention', since the expression could mean part of normal health care practice such as giving patients information about their illness. See the example of giving information as an intervention in the *OTPM*.[34]

A second, and different kind of point, is that even if there were evidence that the close relationship with the professional solved the patient's distress, it still would not be possible to achieve. The reason is that it would require resources of professional time which are not available except for a small minority of patients. It is the case that only a minority of people dying, even in the United Kingdom where specialist palliative care is well developed, receive care from a specialist team, let alone a psychiatrist or psychotherapist as advocated by some authorities.[35,36] If it is the professionals' duty to solve patients' psychosocial and spiritual problems, then they are bound to fail. In reality, it makes no sense to say that doctors and nurses have obligations and responsibilities which they cannot possibly fulfil.

Our third and basic point however is that normal human emotions and reactions should not be medicalized. Personal relationships and personal emotions cannot be translated into symptoms which require professional management. This point is made very powerfully by Christopher Cherry. He explains that, in the context of a managed health care system, the patient matters simply because he or she is a human being. The patient does not matter in a personal sense to the professional, for the personal attributes and qualities of the patient, which he calls 'the particularities of identity', are valued in the context of personal relationships, rather than in the patient/professional relationship necessary in such a system. He states:

> Ideas such as love, devotion, caring for, suffering with, feeling compassion for and empathizing with are most at home where there is minimal abstraction from identity, where alleviation of misery, deprivation, sickness and suffering falls within the frame of a pre-existing relationship which has started and developed independently and of which it cannot therefore be the point. Where such issues are the sole reason for a relationship the moral epistemic concepts are significantly modified; a modification which amounts, in essence, to an abstraction from identity [...]
>
> [Professional] carers and writers on caring often give themselves a bad time because they mistake what is a logical impossibility for a shortfall in compassion. They do not adequately distinguish between the relief of suffering as something called for within the course of a relationship of which that suffering is just one feature and the relief of suffering as the essence of a relationship, as the only reason why it should be there at all. With this goes a failure to distinguish between the logics of "non-abstracted" and "abstracted" caring, and hence a sense that if only they tried hard enough they could offer the first and not merely the second.

He goes on to state that:

> This value (non-abstracted caring) cannot conceivably exist within a managed health care system, although it can of course co-exist - in the community, for example—with other values the system incorporates or generates. At the same time, many who believe in the centrality of this non-transferable value believe also that its unavoidable

> sacrifice is a price regularly (and increasingly) worth paying for the institutional goods and professional skills the system makes possible.[37]

His argument is convincing. From it and the above discussion one must conclude that the close personal relationship which the philosophy of palliative care advocates to the end of relieving psychosocial and spiritual distress is neither achievable nor desirable. 'Non-abstracted' caring, which is caring on a personal level with the degree of intimacy which it requires, is not an appropriate end in a managed health care system.

The very provision of palliative care services carries an emotionally important message to patients about their value to the rest of the community. Cherry makes this point in a footnote, where he comments that people want to know why it should be thought worthwhile to try to make them better, and that they may also care about who makes this happen.

Experience in palliative care shows that patients are touched by the fact that the community continues to provide for their needs, even if inadequately, when clearly there is no prospect of recovery or return to what might be regarded as a useful and productive life. It matters to them, and in some way consoles them, that members of the community are willing to fund their care, either charitably as an extra to the NHS provision, or by taxation via NHS services in the UK for example. Charitable provision is arguably an even stronger indication to patients that their community still considers their welfare important, and it is interesting to note that even NHS specialist palliative care services are to some extent reliant on charitable provision.

It may be that the provision of care for these patients by the community demonstrates to them that they are in some way valued, even if that is an 'abstracted' value in the sense that the community must value them as human beings and cannot value them in a personal sense. It seems to follow that being valued by one's community enables one to retain a sense of self-respect in illness, which must be essential to well-being. Howard Brody, in his book *Stories of sickness*, comments that self-respect is fundamentally a social concept—it relies on social reciprocity. He further explains that self-respect is an attribute of persons that figures centrally in how they respond to sickness. In order to maintain their self-respect they need affirmation of their altered life-plans by others, and those chronically sick or handicapped 'need a very strong and repetitive symbolic reassurance from the state that their lives are viewed by their fellow citizens as being worth living'.[38] The provision of specialist palliative care provides this reassurance from the community.

Let us return to Dame Cicely Saunders' well known comment—'you matter because you are you, and you matter until the last moment of your life'.[39] If we interpret these words as meaning that the patient matters to the community and so is cared for via health care professionals, then this interpretation makes sense in the context of a publicly funded health care system. The patient, abstracted from his or her actual identity, matters to the community which demonstrates this by providing care. The health care professionals are the agents of the community's care for its members. In contrast it is much less plausible to say that the particular patient is cared for in a 'non-abstracted' sense by the particular health care professional. This latter interpretation, popular as it is amongst specialists in palliative care, is unrealistic, and if it were lived out in practice would probably lead to harm both to patients and staff.

The first question we asked in this chapter on psychosocial care was whether doctors and nurses should seek to control the patient's psychological and social and spiritual problems as part of their remit. Since this requires the establishment of a close personal relationship which we have concluded is morally undesirable, then either an alternative way to achieve the goal must be achieved, or we have to conclude that the goal as stated is unacceptable, and so must either be abandoned or be modified in some way. Rather than modifying or abandoning the goal, it is often suggested that the patient's psychological and social problems can be resolved by the introduction of another kind of professional relationship. This relationship is very different from the traditional doctor-patient or nurse-patient relationship, but it is still a special relationship. It is that which occurs between 'counsellor' and 'client'.

7.1.5 An alternative: the client-counsellor relationship

The last twenty years has seen a rapid rise in the popularity of 'counselling' as a way of dealing with human distress, traumatic life events, or difficulties with relationships. As such, it has everything to do with psychosocial care, and perhaps something to do with spiritual care if the latter is taken as helping a person in a search for meaning. Thus it is often advocated as a way of helping the dying. In the context of palliative care it is said to have two objectives: 'first, to identify accurately the key concerns of patients and carers, whether they be physical, social, psychological, or spiritual in nature; second, to help patients and carers find strategies to resolve those concerns that can be resolved or adapt to those that cannot'.[40]

Counselling occurs in the context of a well-defined relationship which has a contractual basis. It is now said to be a set of skills which can be (and it is argued should be) taught. It is not a relationship which naturally evolves between people, so that counsellors have to be trained to fulfil their role (and clients have to agree to their role). Thus courses for professional counsellors are available, and increasingly similar courses are recommended for health care professionals.

The meaning of the term 'counselling' has become blurred by its many different uses. In many contexts the term is reserved for a highly specialized relationship, initially recommended by Carl Rogers who founded the 'non-directive' school of counselling in the 1950s. This specialized relationship is characterized by three attitudes which are fundamental to the counsellor's role; respect, empathy, and genuineness. In addition, it is recommended that the counsellor practices within a recognized 'code of ethics' which is peculiar to this one relationship. The code comprises principles which are summarized as follows by Parkes, Relf, and Couldrick in their book on counselling in terminal care and bereavement: 'Counselling should be practised within a recognized code of ethics. It should: be focused, with specific goals; move towards the client's autonomy; be time limited; be a one-way relationship; involve explicit agreement that the client is working towards change; be supported by a programme of training; and be supervised'.[41]

These authors give helpful explanations regarding the application of these principles in the context of palliative care. The client (more traditionally the patient) must explicitly agree to be working towards change, and that change or goal would be a change in his/her perception of his/her situation. Thus the goal of the counselling process would be to decrease the patient's perception of isolation or hopelessness. The counselling process, in moving towards the client's autonomy, allows the client to gain more control over his/her situation. Since it is a one-way relationship, the counsellor's personal experiences or standards should not normally be divulged to the client.

Whilst these authors do stress that the relationship with the *bereaved* must be time-limited, entailing negotiation of duration and frequency of sessions, they also acknowledge that this principle 'may be difficult to put into practice and may even be inappropriate' with *patients*, not least because time is necessarily limited by the progression of the disease towards death.[42]

In contrast, Maguire and Pitceathly in the *OTPM* note that 'patients and carers need to be orientated to the goals of counselling, the duration, and likely number of sessions'.[43] Thus the counsellor sees the patient for pre-arranged sessions lasting for a set time. This is not an open-ended, flexible relationship, but is clearly contractual. Whereas in health care a patient is frequently permitted to take more time than the allocated outpatient clinic appointment, and patients are free to ask for help when they feel they need it, in counselling the schedule of meetings is agreed in advance and the client is expected to adhere to it as a foundation of the relationship. Access to the counsellor is therefore certainly not based on client-perceived need.

Maguire and Piceathly comment that this measure is necessary to protect the health care professional from unrealistic expectations of patients or their families, and also to reduce the risk of health care professionals becoming over-involved, and devaluing the ability of patients and carers to find effective ways of coping using their own resources. This structure to the relationship contrasts sharply with the close personal relationship usually advocated between patients and professionals in palliative care, as already described. Readers of the *OTPM* might reasonably be confused regarding the nature of the relationship which they ought to have with their patients, since some authors stress close involvement whereas those describing counselling stress the necessity for professional detachment.

The idea of the specialized relationship is that the counsellor will help the client find the solution to the client's problems, or will help the client to resolve the issue which is causing distress. However, the responsibility for working on the problem definitely lies with the client - the counsellor is regarded as having a facilitative role only. This means that the counsellor cannot be held responsible for the outcome of the relationship. This is in contrast to health care, where a professional is held accountable for the outcome of treatment.

So far we have summarized the principles underlying counselling, and noted the three attitudes fundamental to the counselling role, namely respect, empathy and genuineness. We must now consider whether experts instructing health care professionals regarding best practice in palliative care believe that the counsellor/client relationship should be adopted generally by health care professionals towards the patients and their relatives.

Parkes *et al.* recommend that health care professionals use counselling, according to the principles and fundamental attitudes described above, as one 'helping strategy' in the care of patients. They regard it as a strategy in which the patient/client 'has greater control and the professional plays a more enabling role'.[44] They contrast this with other helping strategies, such as direct action (treatment), and giving advice, information, and reassurance, which they regard as fitting the general ethos of health care. In these strategies they see the professional as more in control.

When counselling is described as just one strategy, in a spectrum of strategies used by professionals to help people, one might conclude that these authors are suggesting that health care professionals move in and out of the counsellor/client relationship with patients and relatives. According to this model, professionals would sometimes adopt the more traditional attitudes and principles of health care, for example in giving advice, information and reassurance and in directly intervening in the patient's life by active treatment following consent. At other times they would switch into the specialized counselling relationship, adopting its principles and attitudes.

But this idea of switching from one relationship to another is precisely *not* what these authors are suggesting. Instead, they state that 'basic counselling skills' are essential to asses patients' needs, and that the ability to asses these needs is fundamental to all the helping strategies.[45] It follows that health care professionals must learn and practise these counselling skills in order to pursue any helping strategy.

The authors do acknowledge that during the learning process 'we usually go through a period of feeling de-skilled and self-conscious in our interactions with others'. But they claim that 'these feelings of self-consciousness fade as the new techniques become internalized and the end result is likely to be a major improvement in both skills and confidence'.[46]

Thus the authors are actually recommending that the attitudes and behaviours of the counsellor/client relationship should be not just learned but rather 'internalized'. But what does it mean to 'internalize' a set of attitudes and behaviours? It must mean that they would come to pervade and dominate our interactions with people in general. In other words, what would have been spontaneous and genuine reactions would be replaced by trained and artificial responses. This would have a major impact on *all* our relationships. The authors may regard this as a good thing—but few people outside of the counselling ideology would agree with them. For the purposes of our present discussion this recommendation, if followed in practice, would mean that the traditional principles and attitudes of health care would be abandoned in favour of the principles and attitudes of the specialized counselling relationship.

At the same time the authors do acknowledge that 'the majority of patients and relatives seldom seek formal counselling from qualified counsellors but many want to talk over their circumstances with their professional carers'. No wonder! They go on to note that: 'in palliative care, counselling usually takes place within the context of a relationship which is primarily focused on non-counselling activities'.[47] Despite recognizing that patients and relatives are not seeking the relationship of client to counsellor in their contact with health care professionals the authors effectively instruct professionals that the role of counsellor, with its associated principles, attitudes, and behaviours, must be adopted generally with patients and relatives. Furthermore, the key attitudes must be *conveyed* to the patient or relative by behaviours called 'communication skills' if the patient or relative 'is to feel understood'.[48]

In the *OTPM* chapter on 'Learning Counselling' by Maguire and Pitceathly, the term 'counselling' seems to be used to describe a relationship with the patient and family which health care professionals would recognize as being similar to the usual relationship of professional to patient advocated for palliative care.[49] But there are crucial differences, in terms of clearer temporal boundaries to the interaction, limitation of emotional involvement by the professional, and learned techniques and responses by the professional. Thus these authors also recommend that professionals adopt the principles, attitudes, and behaviours of the counsellor in their relationships with patients and relatives.

It cannot be over-emphasized that these principles, attitudes, and behaviours—perhaps summed up by the word 'detachment'—are totally incompatible with the principles, attitudes and behaviours more typically recommended in palliative care—best summed up by the word 'involvement'. They cannot be combined. Moreover, switching from one to the other (even were it possible) would produce confusion and distress in anyone, far less a terminally ill patient or bereaved relative. We shall now discuss the three concepts which are central to the theory of counselling: empathy, respect, and genuineness.

(a) Empathy

Parkes *et al.* state that: 'Empathy involves being able to sense accurately and appreciate another person's reality and to convey that understanding sensitively'.[50] Thus empathizing has two components. The first is the ability to understand and share the emotions of the other person so as to enter his/her experiential world. The second is to behave in such a way that the client (or patient/relative) becomes persuaded that one has achieved this level of understanding. They quote Carl Rogers' definition of empathetic listening, which leaves the reader in no doubt about the level of understanding which is expected to be achieved by the counsellor:

> It [emphathic listening] means entering the private perceptual world of the other and becoming thoroughly at home in it. It involves being sensitive, moment by moment, to the changing meanings which flow in this other person, to the fear or rage or tenderness or confusion or whatever, that he or she is experiencing. It means temporarily living in the other's life, moving about in it delicately without making judgements. It's a way of saying "I'm with you, I've been listening carefully to what you've been saying and expressing and I'm checking to see if my understanding is accurate".[51]

It should be noted here that having entered the experiential world of the other person the counsellor must not make any judgements—this non-judgemental component is fundamental to the attitude of respect which we discuss later.

The problems of empathy are closely linked to those of compassion already described. By listening to the client's story and interpretation of events, the counsellor is expected to empathize with the client. But empathy entails understanding the meaning that emotions and experience have for the other person. It is doubtful if even very close friends or spouses can achieve this level of understanding, so it seems literally incredible that it could be achieved by a counsellor listening to the client for a few fixed (and often fee-paying) sessions. The root problem is that it is not clear whether 'empathy' means an end state in which one has achieved an understanding of what the client is experiencing, or whether 'empathy' is a process of trying to understand it. This lack of clarity is illustrated by phrases from texts on counselling such as 'The use of empathy also signals that the health professional is trying to understand the patients' or carers' reactions'.[52]

There is also a fundamental ambiguity at the heart of understanding another person's experience. Are we understanding what the other person might be feeling or thinking, or what we might feel or think in the same situation? The official answer is no doubt that we are trying to understand what the other person is feeling. But how is it possible, even in principle, to know that what we are 'understanding' is the other person's feelings, as distinct from imagining what our own might be in the situation?

In the context of palliative care it seems particularly unlikely that the counsellor can really understand the client's feelings regarding the terminal illness. Understanding of this kind usually requires having had a similar experience, as is shown in the popularity of self-help groups. The counsellor is very unlikely to have had any personal experience of receiving a fatal diagnosis, nor of the reality of confronting death in the near future, nor of the weakness and exhaustion the illness may bring, nor of the depression which afflicts many patients at some time. Without such understanding the counsellor cannot possibly enter the experiential world of the patient. So perhaps the goal of empathy, even if desirable, is unattainable.

Despite this obvious problem, it is thought to be important that the client is convinced that the counsellor is listening and empathizes. To this end the counsellor is told to adopt certain non-verbal behaviours such as postures towards the client, positions for chairs, level heights for conversation, amounts of eye contact, and even mirroring behaviour such as smiling when the client smiles. Verbally, the counsellor is expected to keep reflecting back to the client the last phrase of sentences or a paraphrase of what the client has said. Alternatively, the counsellor may be trained to give frequent summaries of what has been said. This is intended to demonstrate that the counsellor is listening and that the client has been 'heard and understood', and it also allows the client to clarify his statement and to correct misunderstandings.[53] The counsellor is also expected to demonstrate empathy by statements such as 'that must have been difficult/awful for you'.

The problem with such trained behaviour is that it is easily recognized as such, and when so recognized the client may (quite reasonably) lose faith in the genuineness of the counsellor. Those supporting the use of counselling say that the repetition of phrases gives encouragement to the client, like a soft reflective mirror, but clients may feel that they are speaking to a rock face and hearing the echo.

The aspects of counselling associated with achieving empathy have, perhaps unfortunately, been described as a set of skills called 'listening skills', 'active listening', or 'communication skills' which many health care professionals have now been taught. Our concern is that those health care professionals who truly gave patients their full attention, in the Asklepian sense, would naturally and genuinely have communicated that attention to their patients. They would have encouraged and enabled patients to tell their story. The quality of their interaction with the patient would not have been improved by a 'communication skills' course. Indeed, it might have been adversely affected as they became distracted by intrusive awareness of their own verbal and non-verbal behaviour, as they inhibited their own natural responses, and as they consciously adopted trained responses instead. Those who were not good communicators or did not truly give patients their attention in the Asklepian sense may or may not have been helped by being taught communication skills or listening skills—the worst but quite likely possibility is that they come to sound to the patient like a patronizing computer programme.

Our view is that health care professionals should simply be encouraged to give their full attention to the patient, in the Asklepian sense. Ironically, this sort of attention is well described by Parkes *et al.* in their section on active listening:

> This demands giving people our total attention. It is not a passive process but an active engagement. It requires the use of all our senses. It means listening with our ears to what is being said and to the tone of voice, listening with our minds to understand the message contained in the words, listening with our eyes to what is being conveyed through the client's posture, bearing, and gestures, and listening with our hearts to the human being we are trying to understand. Listening in this way enables clients to feel that we are really there with them and value who they are.[54]

But surely it will be impossible for the vast majority of people to give their whole attention to the patient in this way if there is trained conscious awareness of our own and the patient's non-verbal behaviour, of the need to reflect back or paraphrase what the patient has just said, or of the need to mirror the patient's facial expression. If all these factors are also in our minds, how can we genuinely 'be there with the patient'?

We would argue that the stress should be upon the attention given to what the patient is trying to convey, rather than upon stereotyped behaviours and manipulative ways of conveying the impression that the client is being 'understood and valued'.

The authors state that 'the need for attention becomes acutely pertinent as the end of life approaches'.[55] If this is the case, then our aim should be to give patients our attention, rather than to appear to do so. If we focus on the latter, we cannot also do the former. And in failing to give patients our attention we will probably miss factors vitally important in our professional role of relieving physical symptoms and giving patients the information they seek.

(b) Respect

The attitude of respect, as described in the role of the counsellor, is problematic in that it entails being non-judgemental. This component was stressed by Rogers.[56] Being non-judgemental is sometimes also referred to as giving the client 'unconditional positive regard'.

Of respect, Parkes *et al.* state that: 'The aim is to convey our belief that each person is worthwhile, unique and valuable'. They note that we convey respect by 'not making snap judgements or by being critical' and by 'encouraging clients to make their own decisions rather than assuming that we know best'.[57] But a non-judgemental attitude, or one which offers unconditional positive regard, is not the normal attitude of one person to another. It is morally problematic in any relationship, and it entails particular problems in the context of the health care professional relationship to patients or their relatives.

Thus if the counsellor (or health care professional) is truly intellectually non-judgemental as well as verbally non-judgemental then the counsellor must hold no personal values, or at least must not believe that any particular way of living and dying is any better than another. The counsellor must be a post-modernist. But most health care professionals working with terminally ill patients do believe that some ways of living and dying are better than others. For example, they do seem to believe that peaceful acceptance of death is better than bitter striving against it or denial (Section 7.1.2 above). They tend to regard the healing of fraught relationships as preferable to dying with ongoing family tensions and strife. Health care professionals from their experience will know that some ways of living the end of one's life seem to give rise to greater distress than others. Thus health care professionals, and even professional counsellors, are very unlikely to be non-judgemental intellectually.

Of course it might be argued that whilst professionals will inevitably have their own views and values regarding better and worse ways of dying they should not express those views verbally. Certainly in the traditional doctor or nurse-patient relationship the professional inhibits any desire to tell patients what they may think of the way the latter conduct their relationships and religious lives. On the other hand they have a professional duty to inform patients of lifestyles which are injurious to health, and they may even have a duty to try to get patients to change those lifestyles. They certainly have a duty not to provide treatments which will cause overall harm to the patient rather than benefit. But such a duty is almost certainly incompatible with encouraging patients 'to make their own decisions rather than assuming we know best' in the context of deciding what treatment options should be offered to patients.

Yet in the context of the counsellor/client relationship the counsellor should not be verbally judgmental of the patient's way of living and dying, however injurious to himself or those around him. This is in contrast to both the professional/patient relationship and close personal relationships. The counselling role is, in this sense, very passive. Moreover, since in this regard it does not resemble any relationships which have evolved naturally in society it is also artificial. People will not behave naturally in a totally non-judgmental way— they will have to be trained to do so.

Consistency requires that the non-judgmental counsellor should also be non-directive towards the client. This concept is a cornerstone of counselling. The counsellor must not tell the client what he or she 'ought' to do. Indeed, the counsellor must guard against giving any such hints to the client, leaving the latter to work it out for himself.

Thus, if health care professionals are to adopt the attitude of respect as defined in the counselling role, they would have to be trained out of their professional role of giving advice and reassurance, and into a new non-directive role where the patient alone determines (and presumably takes responsibility for) his own treatment plan. This is another example of the total incompatibility between the attitude and approach of the palliative care professional and the counsellor. The former is committed to certain values whereas the latter attempts to be value-free.

(c) Genuineness

Regarding genuineness, Parkes *et al.* state:

> The aim is to be ourselves in the relationship and thereby convey that we have a genuine concern and can be trusted.[58]

They stress that we convey we are genuine by responding naturally, not pretending to be someone that we are not, being spontaneous, and by making sure that our expressions and bodily gestures are congruent with what we are saying.

The term 'congruence' requires some explanation. One person is said to be congruent with another when he is accurately aware of what he is experiencing, and when he communicates to another fully and honestly exactly what he is experiencing. In counselling, congruence is thought to be a good thing for people. It is seen as a goal for the client, and so presumably also for the counsellor.

There are several difficulties with this idea. Firstly, it is not always possible to be sure what one is thinking or experiencing in a given situation because our motives and emotions can be complex and inaccessible. Secondly, if congruence is 'being what you are' at all levels of feeling and awareness, and then communicating that to another, then there is surely a risk of bringing a relationship (of whatever nature) to an abrupt, unsatisfactory and possibly destructive end. People would need to be deeply attached at a personal level to withstand the full blast of congruence! In the context of the relationship between the patient and the health care professional it would not be acceptable to be congruent, since this might entail expressing strong disapproval, inappropriate affection, or worse still sexual attraction!

It must follow that it is impossible to be both non-judgemental, non-directive and yet congruent at the same time. One would have to be a true post-modernist, fully committed to the view that no one way of living and dying is any better than another, in order to be genuinely non-judgemental and non-directive with a client. This view is not compatible with being a health care professional, for the latter certainly do (and should) have views about ways of living and dying which are most compatible with health.

Yet Parkes *et al.* state that being genuine 'does not mean putting aside our role as a doctor, social worker or nurse but being ourselves within that role'.[59] But surely it is not logically possible to remain in our professional role, and at the same time adopt the incompatible attitude of being steadfastly non-judgemental and non-directive towards patients and their relatives. Nor is it logically possible simultaneously to practise trained verbal and non-verbal behaviours that convey respect and empathy, ensure that our own non-verbal behaviour is congruent with what we are saying, and yet respond 'naturally' and 'spontaneously', and be 'ourselves in the relationship'. No amount of training could enable health care professionals to adopt and sustain such conflicting roles and behaviours, nor could it enable them to respond 'genuinely' whilst they struggled to do so. These policies are logically incompatible.

More worrying still is the emphasis on 'conveying' to the patient that 'we have a genuine concern and can be trusted'. Once again, it seems that professionals are being encouraged and trained to produce a set of behaviours which will give the patient or relative the impression that our concern is genuine and that we can be trusted. This endeavour appears highly manipulative particularly since its practice is anything but genuine. And what is it that we 'can be trusted' to do, as health care professionals forced into the artificial role and relationship of 'counsellor' to patients and their relatives, who in turn have been forced into the role and relationship of 'client'?

This description of the central precepts of counselling leads us to two conclusions. The first is that it seems logically impossible to combine these concepts and associated 'counselling skills' in any human relationship. The second is that it is morally unacceptable to attempt to introduce them into the professional/patient relationship of palliative care. Indeed, patients would probably be harmed by health care professionals becoming enmeshed in role conflicts through attempting to be a counsellor. In order to pursue counselling both the patient and the health care professional would have to change roles, and this is simply not a practical possibility. Therefore, the artificial relationship of counselling should be rejected as a method for health care professionals to solve the psychological, social and spiritual problems of their patients. Counselling should not be regarded as a way to achieve this goal.

7.2 Psychosocial and spiritual care: an alternative approach

In an earlier version of the WHO philosophy it was said that the aim was to 'control' the patient's psychological, social, and spiritual problems.[60] It is right that this aim has been abandoned. The idea of 'controlling' such problems is deeply counter-intuitive, principally because it hints of brainwashing and is certainly destructive and disrespectful of the patient's autonomy. Furthermore, it is exceedingly unlikely that health care professionals could ever attain this undesirable goal, since they cannot meet the patient's psychosocial and spiritual needs; and the participation of patients themselves is essential in relieving such problems—no technical solution administered by professionals and received by patients could ever be successful. The attempt to 'control' another person's psychological, emotional and spiritual problems represents Hippocratic medicine at its least appealing, and it is astonishing that in palliative medicine the idea could ever have gained currency.

In the current version of the WHO philosophy, 'control' has been replaced by 'impeccable assessment and treatment.of pain and other problems, physical, psychosocial and spiritual'. The arrogance implied by the word 'control' has been abandoned, but there is no difference in substance—the patient's psychosocial and spiritual problems are still being identified in the Hippocratic language of mainstream medicine, and are open to the objections we have already raised.

This leaves us with the question of whether the goal should be completely abandoned. In that case a policy could be adopted whereby health care professionals see the patient's emotional, social and spiritual state as strictly the patient's affair, and they cease trying to address any problems which patients might raise. Obviously, answers to enquiries about the illness and its likely progress, together with realistic reassurance to counter fears should always be given.

This solution seems excessively restrictive. For professionals will always want to try to alleviate the emotional distress of patients, and from their experience they will have learned that certain approaches to other patients and families proved helpful in similar circumstances. This is not to say that there is a professional skill in alleviating the patient's emotional distress, but simply to say that professional experience combined with ordinary human contact can be used to alleviate such distress. In other words, professionals can use their common humanity to comfort the patient, through companionship, in combination with giving advice based on the relevant professional knowledge of similar situations.

Thurstan Brewin has termed this sort of professional contact 'friendly professional interest' or FPI. He believes:

> In a "hopeless" situation, tender loving care is not enough, concern and compassion are not enough. Somewhere along the road between old-fashioned TLC and new-fangled counselling, lies something as old as Medicine itself, which I have called here friendly professional interest. For the doctor—whatever else is said or done—FPI is the basic minimum. It need not take up a lot of time; and it does not need special training beyond what ought to be given in every Medical School. Lack of it is a common cause of low morale and misery.[61]

He recommends a regular but informal visit, probably lasting only a few minutes, and perhaps as little as once a week. He stresses that the professional's approach should be easy, friendly, yet interested and professional. He is not recommending that the professionals step out of role, but rather that they should strive for certain qualities. Of professional friendliness he says:

> The ability of one person to lend strength to another (not just in medicine, but also in the way that a good leader does, for example when men or women face possible death in some other kind of threat or disaster) is a mystery that nobody entirely understands. But, for my money, in medical situations—especially advanced cancer—just being natural and friendly has a lot to do with it. Look at the way some hospital cleaners and porters boost the morale of frightened patients. Do they have special understanding, spiritual inspiration, or powers of leadership? Not usually. How many communication and counselling courses have they attended? None. They are just natural and relaxed, with friendly good humour and no awkwardness or embarrassment [...]

> Professional friendship is not quite the same as ordinary friendship, but much that applies still holds true. A friend is warm and welcoming at each meeting. A friend pays small compliments. A friend has at least some idea of how the patient feels; some idea of what she has been going through; understands how her moods may vary (maybe hope one day, despair the next). A friend listens; knows the value of a little praise; asks how she can help. A friend is just as ready to talk seriously (if that is what the patient wants) as to joke or gossip. A really supportive friend doesn't go over the top emotionally, but is always concerned; doesn't stay too long; knows when to be silent; doesn't ask too many questions. A doctor should follow suit.[62]

This powerful extract really says it all. Patients want doctors who are genuinely concerned and understanding, as a friend might be, not those who have simply been trained to look concerned and understanding. Courses on counselling and communication skills cannot teach the attitude and qualities that Thurstan Brewin is describing.

At the same time the patient must be able to remain confident in the professionals' competence. Brewin stresses the importance of continuing to examine patients rather than relying exclusively on investigation results. For gentle and respectful but business-like and efficient examination, besides yielding clinical information, stresses to patients:

> that they have not been abandoned, that the doctor is still anxious not to miss anything that could be corrected or prevented. And there is also a chance to lay firm, calm, caring, unhurried hands on all parts of the body, blending professional efficiency with the age-old power of touch to give comfort; at the same time giving a clear signal to the patient that we don't think of him as in any way repugnant, unclean or infectious.[63]

It is important to stress that doctors ought not to be less interested in patients because a diagnosis has been made and the prognosis is very poor, so that cure cannot be offered. Brewin also suggests that professionals should be interested in the patient as a person—most have some events in their lives which are of importance and general interest, and interests in patients as people often leads to increased respect for them.

Howard Brody, in *Stories of sickness*, explains further how ordinary professional contact in listening carefully to the patient's story can help patients and professionals to understand the meaning of the illness for the patient. For the meaning of the illness has much to do with spirituality, and peace of mind for the patient and self-respect. He explains that:

> being sick includes experiencing a special and generally very frightening sort of disruption in the unity of body and self, and it also includes undergoing an alteration in one's social role and in the way one relates to others and vice versa. It is unlikely that these essential features of the sickness story will be elicited by the standard medical

history, but they may be better understood if the patient is asked to relate the meaning he attaches to the illness.[64]

In his foreword to *Narrative based medicine*, he states that 'Some of medicine works extrememly well precisely because it treats people as being all the same; and some of medicine works very well because it treats people as all being different'.[65] His point could be expanded as follows. In both clinical medicine and ethics we must appreciate both the similarities between cases and the differences between them, hence the relevance of casuistry (see Chapter 1, Section 1.8, p. 14). Working out in what way cases are the same and also being aware of their uniqueness and the differences between them is crucial to both casuistry and clinical medicine. The patient's unique story is part of the case history, in fact it is evidence. Furthermore, it goes beyond straight factual evidence because it usually contains insights into the meaning of the illness for the patient.

Howard Brody explains that doctors, in the course of their normal work, can make the meaning of the illness more positive for the patient in three ways:

> First, the illness experience must be given an explanation of the sort that will be viewed as acceptable, given the patient's existing belief system and worldview. Second, the patient must perceive that he or she is surrounded by and may rely upon a group of caring individuals. Third, the patient must achieve a sense of mastery or control over the illness experience, either by feeling personally powerful enough to affect the course of events for the better or by feeling that his or her individual powerlesness can be compensated by the power of some member or members of the caring group (such as the physician).[66]

He is sceptical as to whether courses on ethics can make doctors more compassionate, and considers instead that doctors should be taught always to listen to the patient's story with 'the air of one trying to recognize—trying to make a link between their own humanity and the humanity of the anguished individual before them'.[67] He suggests that this practice should be encouraged in ordinary medical education, and should be integral to clinical work.

In conclusion, it should be noted that our discussion of the WHO philosophy of palliative care as it applies to the psychosocial and spiritual states of our patients has two sides to it. Our negative criticisms are directed at the attempt to carry over the complexities and techniques of Hippocratic medicine from the area of the physical, where they are in the main successful, to the psychosocial, where they are both unsuccessful and inhumane. Our positive suggestions are to the effect that the psychosocial, emotional and spiritual side to a patient's experience should not be ignored, but it does not require either 'control' or 'assessment' and 'treatment'. It requires the kind word, the

Asklepian direct gaze, of the friendly professional. In other words, whatever the complexities of pain relief, this side of palliative care requires something much simpler—the mature and friendly professional.

7.3 **Conclusions**

1 Patients' consent should be sought to in depth questioning and interventions regarding their psychosocial and spiritual welfare.

2 A close personal relationship between patient and professional is potentially harmful to both, unachievable and not sustainable. It is morally undesirable.

3 The requirement for the development of a close personal relationship between patient and professional should not be part of the philosophy of palliative care, nor should the development of the client/counsellor relationship be advocated.

4 The goal of controlling the patient's psychological, social, and spiritual problems, or of assessing and treating them, should be abandoned.

5 It should be replaced by the idea of alleviating those problems within the context of the traditional professional/patient relationship, using ordinary human interaction, sensitive explanations and advice based on professional knowledge and experience, and friendly professional interest.

References

1 WHO (2002). *National cancer control programmes: policies and managerial guidelines*, 2nd edn. WHO, Geneva.

2 Saunders, C. (1972). The care of the dying patient and his family. *Contact*, 38: 12–18.

3 Payne, R., Gonzales, G.R., and Foley, K.M. (2004). The management of pain. In: *Oxford textbook of palliative medicine*, 3ed edn, ed. D. Doyle, G. Hanks, N. Cherny *et al*. Oxford University Press, Oxford: pp.288-315.

4 Vachon, M. (2004a). The emotional problems of the patient in palliative medicine. In: *OTPM*, 3rd edn, op.cit. p. 961.

5 Saunders, C. (1993). Foreword to *Oxford Textbook of Palliative Medicine*, 1st edn, ed. Doyle, D. Hanks, G., MacDonald, N. Oxford University Press, Oxford: pp.v-viii.

6 Saunders, C. (1993). op. cit. p.X.

7 Scott, A. (1998). Nursing, narrative and the moral imagination. In: *Narrative based medicine*, ed. T. Greenhalgh and B. Hurwitz. BMJ Books, London: p. 152.

8 Tschudin, V. (1993). *Ethics in nursing*. Butterworth, London: p.1

9 Churchill, L. (1977). Ethical issues of a profession in transition. *American Journal of Nursing*, 77(5): 873-5.

10 Nouwen, H.J., McNeill, D.P., and Morrison. D.A. (1982). *Compassion*. Darton, Longman & Todd, London.

11 Tschudin, V. (1993). op. cit. p. 10.

12 Wright, E.B., Holcombe, C., and Salmon, P. (2004). Doctors' communication of trust, care, and respect in breast cancer: a qualitative study. *BMJ*, 328: 865.

13 Vachon, M. (2004b). The stress of professional caregivers. In: *OTPM*, 3rd edn, op.cit. pp. 997–8.

14 Cherry, C. (1997). Health care, human worth and the limits of the particular. *Journal of Medical Ethics*, **23**: 310–14.

15 Speck, P., Higginson, I., and Addington-Hall, J. (2004). Spiritual needs in health care. *BMJ*, **329**: 123–4.

16 Fallowfield, L. (2004). Communication with the patient and family in palliative medicine. In: *OTPM*, 3rd edn, op. cit., p. 105.

17 Vachon, M. (1993). Emotional problems in palliative medicine: patient, family, and professional. In: *OTPM*, 1st edn, op.cit., p. 586.

18 Breitbart, W., Chochinov. H.M., and Passik, S.D. (2004). Psychiatric symptoms in palliative medicine. In: *OTPM*, 3rd edn, op. cit., p. 761.

19 Maguire, P. and Pitceathly, C. (2004). Learning counselling. In: *OTPM*, 3rd edn, op. cit., p. 1176.

20 Cassel, E. (1982). The nature of suffering and the goals of medicine. *New England Journal of Medicine*, **306**: 639–45.

21 Maguire, P. (year). Communication with terminally ill patients and their relatives. In: *Handbook of psychiatric and palliative medicine*, ed. H.M. Chochinov and W. Breitbart. Oxford University Press, New York: pp. 291–301.

22 Hinton, J. (1999). The progress of awareness and acceptance of dying assessed in cancer patients and their caring relatives. *Palliative Medicine*, **13**: 19–35.

23 Vachon, M. (2004a). op. cit., p. 975.

24 WHO (2004). *Better palliative care for older people*. WHO, Geneva: p. 28.

25 Breitbart, W., Chochinov, H.M., and Passik, S.D. (2004). In: *OTPM* 3rd edn, op. cit. p. 747.

26 Breitbart, W., Chochinov, H.M., and Passik, S.D. (2004). In: *OTPM* 3rd edn, op. cit. pp. 750–5.

27 WHO (2004). op cit. p. 28.

28 Scott, A. (1998). op. cit. p. 153.

29 Vachon, M. (2004b). op. cit., p. 998.

30 Vachon, M. (2004b). op. cit., p. 999.

31 Fallowfield, L. (2004). op. cit. p. 105.

32 Breitbart, W., Chochinov. H.M., and Passik, S.D. (2004). op. cit. p. 758.

33 WHO (2004). op cit. p. 27.

34 Vachon, M. (2004a). op. cit., p. 964.

35 Breitbart, W., Chochinov. H.M., and Passik, S.D. (2004). op. cit. p. 747.

36 NICE (2004). *Guidance on improving supportive and palliative care for adults with cancer*. NICE, London: p. 77.

37 Cherrry, C. (1997). op. cit. pp. 310–14.

38 Brody, H. (1987). *Stories of sickness*. Yale University Press, London: pp. 540; 132.

39 Saunders, C. (2003). *Watch with me*. Mortal Press, Sheffield: p. 46.

40 Maguire, P. and Pitceathly, C. (2004). op. cit. p. 1176.

41 Parkes, C.M., Relf, M., and Couldrick, A. (1996). *Counselling in terminal care and bereavement*. BPS Books, Leicester: p. 71.

42 Parkes, C.M., Relf, M., and Couldrick, A. (1996). op. cit. p. 50.

43 Maguire, P. and Pitceathly, C. (2004). op. cit. p. 1180.

44 Parkes, C.M., Relf, M., and Couldrick, A. (1996). op. cit. p. 53.

45 Parkes, C.M., Relf, M., and Couldrick, A. (1996). op. cit. pp. 54–55.

46 Parkes, C.M., Relf, M., and Couldrick, A. (1996). op. cit. p. 60.

47 Parkes, C.M., Relf, M., and Couldrick, A. (1996). op. cit. p. 50.

48 Parkes, C.M., Relf, M., and Couldrick, A. (1996). op. cit. p. 59.

49 Maguire, P. and Pitceathly, C. (2004). op. cit., pp. 1176–82.

50 Parkes, C.M., Relf, M., and Couldrick, A. (1996). op. cit. p. 58.

51 Rogers, C. (1975). An unappreciated way of being. *Counselling Psychologist*, 21: 95–103.

52 Maguire, P. and Pitceathly, C. (2004). op. cit., p. 1177.

53 Maguire, P. and Pitceathly, C. (2004). op. cit., p. 1177.

54 Parkes, C.M., Relf, M., and Couldrick, A. (1996). op. cit. p. 60.

55 Parkes, C.M., Relf, M., and Couldrick, A. (1996). op. cit. p. 60.

56 Rogers, C. (1975). op. cit.

57 Parkes, C.M., Relf, M., and Couldrick, A. (1996). op. cit. p. 58.

58 Parkes, C.M., Relf, M., and Couldrick, A. (1996). op. cit. p. 59.

59 Parkes, C.M., Relf, M., and Couldrick, A. (1996). op. cit. p. 59.

60 WHO (1990). *Cancer pain relief and palliative care.* Report of a WHO Expert Committee, Technical Report Series, 804. WHO, Geneva.

61 Brewin, T. (1996). *The friendly professional.* Eurocommunica Publications, Bognor Regis: pp. 74–9.

62 Brewin, T. (1996). op. cit. p. 76.

63 Brewin, T. (1996). op. cit. p. 77.

64 Brody, H. (1987). op. cit. p. 184.

65 Brody, H. (1987). op. cit. p. xiii.

66 Brody, H. (1987). op. cit. p. 6.

67 Brody, H. (1987). op. cit. p. 183.

8

Resource allocation

Introduction

Palliative care, according to the WHO philosophy, is a complex group of assessments and interventions for both patients and their families, with the aim of improving their quality of life. The philosophy statement describes practice in the specialty of palliative care. In view of its emphasis on psychosocial and spiritual care, and its inclusion of families in its remit, this practice can reasonably be expected to consume significantly more resources, of both manpower and money, than conventional care.

Furthermore, the WHO advocates extending the philosophy of palliative care, and the assessments and interventions of specialist palliative care, to all patients who are terminally ill. Even more strikingly, they have also advocated extension of the practice to patients with life-threatening but curable illness.[1] Such a policy requires justification, since it seems very likely that its enactment would require a shift in resources towards palliative care and away from other areas of health care. Indeed, the health economist Alan Maynard wrote in the *OTPM*: 'Making treatment and care choices within palliative care and between palliative care and the numerous other health areas is little more than an unevaluated social experiment at present'.[2] Whilst some evaluation has been undertaken, we will argue that the 2004 WHO recommendations for the expansion of the current philosophy and practice of palliative care to all patients who are terminally ill or have life-threatening but curable illness in Europe are unjustifiable.

The process whereby available resources are distributed between different areas of health care is called macroallocation. Resources are allocated to different specialties and for different treatments, and so the process requires differentiation between services and treatments. In contrast, the process whereby the benefits of a service or treatment are distributed between individual patients is called microallocation. We will discuss only the issue of macroallocation. A fair macroallocation process implies a distribution system designed to achieve two goals: firstly, the best use of resources by using the most cost-effective measures, and secondly, a just or fair distribution of benefit between individuals.

In many countries specialist palliative care has developed largely as a result of charitably funded initiatives. It has not been planned as an integrated part of health care. Allocation of state funding towards its provision has been erratic. The UK development of specialist palliative care exemplifies this rather haphazard approach. The absence of a distribution system for health care and palliative care in particular results in resource allocation which is greatly influenced by political expediency, pressure groups, and the media. This process, described in the UK by Richard Smith, editor of the *BMJ*, as 'muddling through'[3] is unlikely to achieve the goals of equitable distribution.

In the context of palliative care, the cost-effectiveness of the care recommended by the WHO, and as described in the definition, must be assessed. With reference to investment in palliative care services Maynard commented, 'If (investments) are not cost-effective and the resources could generate greater health benefits to patients elsewhere in the health care system, it is sensible (i.e. efficient) to deprive palliative care of funding. Playing Oliver and demanding "more" will no longer serve the interests of patients in any part of the health care system'.[4] Whilst this view may be unpalatable to specialists in palliative care, the public, and the WHO, he is making the point that palliative care must produce an acceptable amount of benefit for patients in comparison with its costs, and that simply recommending that more and more of it be provided regardless of the cost-effectiveness of its various interventions is not morally defensible. Is there an acceptable basis in ethics for the allocation of funds for palliative care?

8.1 **Needs assessment**

The criterion most often used for allocating resources is called a 'needs assessment'. When the term 'need' is used there are two implications: that the satisfaction of the need is instrumental in enabling a benefit to be brought about, and that because the goal is a benefit there is a moral obligation to meet the need. The idea is that research yields evidence regarding interventions which provide benefit, and assertions that patients and their relatives 'need' those beneficial interventions usually follows. Such assertions in turn imply that there is a moral obligation to provide those interventions. But neither research, nor the assertion that patients and relatives have certain needs, tells us which of those 'needs' ought to be met by the service, or how to balance apparently competing needs when there are insufficient resources to meet them all.

The WHO publication on palliative care, *The solid facts*, exemplifies this problem throughout. In the section on ethical arguments, where it is stated that 'good quality care towards the end of life must be recognized as a basic human right', it repeatedly refers to the right to receive care in accordance with patients' needs:

> All people have a right to receive high quality care during serious illness and to a dignified death free of overwhelming pain and in line with their spiritual and religious needs. Although palliative care originally developed for people with cancer, ethical concerns about fairness, equality and equity require that this standard of care be offered to other people with similar needs.... People vary greatly in their willingness to talk openly about their illness or its prognosis, the needs they wish to acknowledge, the level of symptom control they find acceptable, the interventions they will consider, and whom they wish to care for them.[5]

An earlier statement pertaining to the definition of palliative care states: 'Palliative care should be offered as needs develop and before they become unmanageable'. It goes on to say: 'Palliative care has focused on controlling pain and other symptoms, defining needs around patients and their families, and being flexible about doing what is necessary to help people adapt and cope with their situation'.[6]

This last statement gives the impression that patients and their families 'need' anything which would help them adapt and cope, and implies that health care professionals ought to provide anything which would help them to adapt and cope, since what counts as a health care need is 'defined' around the patient and family. According to this notion, health care professionals ought to organize improved housing, the resolution of family disputes, holidays, or a wide range of other non-health-related benefits because they have been seen as 'needs'. In our view this conclusion is unworkable, and must be rejected. The weakness derives from the wide sense of 'need' involved, as we shall show.

A need arises from a desire or aim to achieve a certain goal; that which is needed is instrumental in achieving the goal. According to the WHO philosophy, the overall goal of palliative care is improved quality of life for patients and families. But we have already discussed the major difficulties inherent in the use of the concept of quality of life (Chapter 2). Maynard, in his discussion of the economics of palliative care in the *OTPM* alludes to the difficulty of measuring the benefit or extent of achievement of the goal.[7] At the same time he stresses the importance of the 'identification, measurement, and valuation of all the relevant benefits' as part of economic evaluation of palliative care. Unfortunately, the endeavour of identifying, measuring, and evaluating the achievement of the explicit goals or desired benefits, as improvements in quality of life, is an insuperable obstacle, as we have already argued.

The WHO appears to be defining 'need' very widely as 'capacity to benefit'. Following this line of reasoning has led it to the conclusion that virtually all patients (other than those with an acute and curable illness) need palliative care. Thus those chronically ill, those of any age with a life-threatening illness and those receiving curative treatment should all have access to, and perhaps receive, palliative care, on the grounds that they would all benefit from it. The WHO is saying that there is a moral 'ought' to extend palliative care very widely in order to meet this 'need'.

But as we have stressed throughout, the practice of palliative care, as described in the WHO philosophy statement, is a very complex intervention directed at all aspects of the patient's and family's well-being. It will consume more resources than conventional care. So extending it to the large proportion of patients receiving health care, as suggested by the WHO, would consume massive resources. Since resources are limited, presumably they would have to be diverted away from provision of life-prolonging treatments and care essential to assist patients with the activities of daily living. We would ask whether this could be justified.

Clearly there is a problem if the term 'need' is used in this all-inclusive manner. The association of a need with a moral obligation to meet such needs leads to the conclusion that a health service (or palliative care service) ought to provide everything from which patients and relatives could benefit. If we were to provide everything which would benefit the health of each individual the responsibilities of the health service, let alone palliative care, would be infinite. Moreover, defining 'need' simply as capacity to benefit leads to the conclusion that any patient who would benefit from specialist palliative care needs it. This appears to be the conclusion of the WHO. In its booklet *Palliative care: the solid facts* it states that: 'Emerging needs of people living with serious chronic illnesses, together with new evidence for the effectiveness of palliative care, mean that it must now be offered more widely and integrated more broadly across the health care services'.[8] It goes on to say that: 'The concept of palliative care as an intervention that can be offered alongside potentially curative treatment must be developed and used to meet the needs of ageing populations, as well as those of younger people and children who experience life-threatening illness'.[9]

We would also ask whether it is possible financially or in terms of manpower, to meet these 'needs'. It is important to note that there cannot logically be a moral obligation to do that which is impossible. It is impossible to provide all the health care, or palliative care, from which patients and relatives could benefit.

If 'capacity to benefit' is accepted as a description of 'need', and thus patients need everything they could benefit from, then the association between a 'need' and the obligation to meet that need must break down, because it is impossible to provide everything that patients would benefit from. So if patients are said to need everything they could benefit from, the moral obligation to provide everything they need can no longer exist. It is likely that many people would be uncomfortable with the notion that patients and their families might have needs which there is no moral obligation for society to meet. This idea is deeply counterintuitive.

The way out of this difficulty is to re-examine the idea of a 'capacity to benefit'. We have argued that the concept of need is instrumental—the satisfaction of a need is required to bring about a goal or benefit. But human beings have inexhaustible capacities to benefit, and there cannot be a moral obligation in a publicly or voluntarily funded service to satisfy every capacity to benefit. In the context of health care, of which palliative care is a part, the benefits must be health benefits. Here we are sympathetic to the narrow definition of 'need' provided by Beauchamp and Childress. According to these authors a need is: 'something without which one will be fundamentally harmed'.[10] In the context of palliative care this definition would clearly imply that a patient needs specialist palliative care if without it he or she is destined to sustain fundamental harm such as moderate or severe pain.

In contrast, it is less clear that a desire to die in a particular place constitutes a need which if not satisfied will fundamentally harm a patient. Yet the WHO attributes great importance to achieving the preferred place of care for the patient, and states that 'Policy-makers should encourage the health services to inquire of people their preference for place of care and death. Meeting individual preferences should be *the ultimate measure of success*'[our italics].[11] They note that studies have found that 75 per cent of people would prefer to die at home. Providing the level of care necessary to satisfy basic care needs, especially where the patient is living alone, would require very great resources as it would probably entail one-to-one care in the patient's home for at least a few days, and frequently for much longer. The Childress and Beauchamp definition would probably not result in the desire to die in one's own home being considered as a 'need', but the WHO clearly consider that it is, and that it is a need which ought to be met.

It is even more debatable whether counselling after the loss of a 'significant other' constitutes a need according to the definition which uses the concept of 'fundamental harm'. Yet the WHO advocates bereavement services, even though it states that 'There is relatively little evidence, however, for [...] the targeting of individuals or the benefit of individual therapy, although these aspects are very difficult to evaluate'.[12] If there is little evidence for benefit from the bereavement services, it is surely impossible to argue that the bereaved have been 'fundamentally harmed' because they did not receive such a service.

This discussion shows that where the distribution of health care services is concerned, whether in relation to specialist or non-specialist palliative care, nothing is settled by simply asserting that patients and families have certain 'needs' and that therefore resources must be directed towards those needs. Furthermore, the concept of 'needs assessment' is much more complex and controversial than has hitherto been acknowledged. Finally, the WHO conclusion that chronically ill patients, and patients of all ages facing life-threatening illness (even if curable) need palliative care (which therefore ought to be provided) must be questioned. The enactment of this recommendation would be likely to require much diversion of resources away from other health care interventions, if palliative care were to be provided according to the WHO philosophy.

The root problem with the WHO position is its assumption that a 'need' is a 'capacity to benefit', where that capacity is understood in an open-ended way. We have argued in Chapters 2, 4, and 7 that these benefits, where they exist, are not health-related. In this context our point is the different one that if the WHO position were implemented it would bankrupt any system of health care.

In fact, the WHO avoids proposing this unfortunate outcome by very much simplifying the range of interventions they advocate for patients dying of illnesses other than cancer. It states that:

> simple measures such as good pain relief, communication, information and coordinated care from skilled professionals are effective in reducing symptoms and suffering. It is unlikely that these experiences differ widely by disease or across countries. This strongly suggests that it is time to make a more active and concerted effort to improve palliative care, concentrating on the implementation of simple effective measures based on the complexity and seriousness of the illness and on the needs of the patient and family.[13]

This down to earth statement seems an entirely sensible conclusion. The problem is that it describes what most of us would understand to be competent health care, not peculiar to palliative care or specialist palliative care. Moreover, this description of health care differs significantly from the philosophy of care described in the WHO philosophy of palliative care plus its associated explanatory section, where much more complex assessment and intervention are suggested. It seems that the WHO is running two different and inconsistent accounts of what should be offered by palliative care. We strongly recommend the simpler and more down to earth account as being workable and affordable.

The recommendations of the WHO are rightly influential, as are those of national bodies making recommendations for the provision of palliative care.

Such documents use the term 'need' frequently and as the basis for the obligation to provide services. The implications of the use of this term reach beyond the confines of small groups of economists and health care professionals. The range of meanings intended by people using the term 'need' easily gives rise not only to confusion, but also to feelings of guilt or resentment among health care practitioners and the public. Because of the strong association between the concept of a health care need and the moral obligation to meet it, health care practitioners are likely to feel guilty if they cannot provide those interventions that they consider their patients need. This guilt is likely to persist whether they consider a need to be something from which a patient might benefit, or something which if not met will lead to a fundamental harm. Health care practitioners may also resent being placed in the situation of having to decide which patients should have their needs met and which should not.

Furthermore, members of the public, especially if themselves ill, are likely to consider that they 'need' those treatments or services from which they would expect to benefit. They are likely to feel resentment or anger when they do not have access to such care, even if the benefit thus denied them is relatively small.

Our recommendation is that in a 'needs assessment' the needs in question should be confined to those which are instrumental in bringing about health-related benefits, where those benefits are ones without which a patient will be fundamentally harmed. They are advisedly described by the WHO in its simpler account of what should be offered as quoted above.[14]

8.2 Efficiency

Achievement of explicit goals is central to discussions regarding efficiency. Economists discuss the meaning of efficiency at great length, but a more pragmatic approach is required for use by those who must distribute health care in the clinical context. Uwe Reinhardt has suggested such a pragmatic interpretation: 'among several policies—*with all of them designed to achieve exactly the same goal*—the most efficient policy is the one that reaches that same specified goal with the least expenditure of real resources (human labor, energy, materials, land and so on)'.[15] His use of italics here emphasizes that efficiency is always directed towards a goal, and that policies or processes can be compared in terms of efficiency *only if* they are all directed towards the same specified goal.

Even when the goals are made explicit, assessing the extent to which they are achieved may be very difficult. This is particularly true in palliative care where it can be very difficult to assess the success of a specialist palliative care service in achieving symptom relief, let alone alleviation of psychological distress. It is then even more difficult to decide whether the specialist service achieved such goals more efficiently than conventional primary and secondary non-specialist care. It is (relatively) easy to sum the human and financial resources entailed by a service or treatment, but much more difficult to assess the extent to which the goal(s) of that service or treatment are met.

Cost-effectiveness is closely related to efficiency. It is very unfortunate for those who have to allocate health care, and particularly specialist palliative care, that effectiveness (the achievement of goals) is so difficult to assess, for it follows that efficiency and cost-effectiveness will also be difficult to assess.

Macro-allocation must entail the comparison of efficiency of services and treatments, but until we have established more explicit goals, and more reliable methods of assessing, even qualitatively, the achievement of those goals, then comparison of services in terms of efficiency is at a very primitive stage. This has been noted by authors writing on evidence-based practice in palliative medicine who note 'Until we have good study methods for individual trials it will remain difficult to draw strong evidence-based conclusions about service delivery and packages of care'.[16]

Given that it is difficult to gain evidence for the effectiveness of palliative care services, it is difficult to ascertain precisely what services should be provided. The WHO states that 'Services should be available on the basis of need in terms of symptoms and problems, and their *effectiveness* in meeting that need, rather than on the basis of diagnosis' [our italics].[17]

Many studies have attempted to assess or measure the impact of specialist palliative care services on patients' and relatives' quality of life, in order to provide information as a basis for future resource allocation and to justify the present existence of such services. Since palliative care philosophy states that the ultimate aim is to improve that quality of life, then it appears essential to evaluate outcome in terms of quality of life. Whilst pain and symptom control are important, evaluating these factors alone is deemed insufficient to prove that palliative care services are capable of achieving what they claim to achieve in terms of improving the quality of life of patients and their families.

In 1999 a systematic literature review of the impact of specialist palliative care services on patients' quality of life was carried out by Salisbury *et al.* Eighty-six papers were reviewed but the overall conclusion was that 'there [was] little robust evidence that any form of organization of specialist palliative care offers significant advantages in terms of impact on the patients' quality of life'. They thought that this negative result might be due to their finding that measurement tools for quality of life 'all have problems and none have yet achieved widespread acceptability'.[18] They also noted significant problems in research in palliative care. Despite these considerable difficulties they concluded that rigorous comparative research should continue in order to provide evidence of improvement in patients' quality of life.

The philosophy of palliative care appears to have chained researchers to the wheel of a task which is unachievable. We would argue that it would be preferable to conduct qualitative research, of a comparative nature, on the impact of specialist palliative care on separate domains of quality of life, for example on pain, mobility and mood. This would be difficult but not logically impossible. If such studies indicated benefit to patients, then that data could be used in forming judgements about resource allocation.

It would be unhelpful to try to combine the evaluation of the domains of quality of life because they are so different in nature that they are incommensurable—they cannot logically be weighed against each other or added to make a single global assessment. A global assessment, even in descriptive terms, simply hides the important changes in separate domains—a service which improved pain control but also managed to increase psychological distress would not be very helpful.

The WHO, in its summary of the role and effectiveness of specialist palliative teams, noted that 'the evidence on the effectiveness of specialist palliative care teams consistently adds up to benefits for patients and families, as measured by the control of pain and other symptoms and the satisfaction expressed by patients and their families'.[19] It noted that the teams usually care for a selected group of patients who have the most complex needs for symptom control, communication, and co-ordination of care. Thus some research, which clearly evaluated specific areas such as symptom control and patient satisfaction, and in a specific group of patients, has shown benefits. It is interesting that the WHO does not claim that evidence has shown that quality of life was improved—a claim which would be much harder (and perhaps impossible) to substantiate.

The lack of evidence of improvement in quality of life from specialist palliative care is crucial if the gain in terms of Quality Adjusted Life Years (QALYs) is considered when funding decisions are made. If it were possible to demonstrate a quality of life improvement resulting from palliative care it is likely that the change would be small, especially as the patients' general condition is usually deteriorating with time. Moreover, an improvement in quality score, say from 0.5 to 0.6, would be of very short duration since patients usually receive such specialist care for only a short time—perhaps only 3 to 6 months, and sometimes only a few weeks.

The combination of an increase in quality of 0.1 (where 1 represents quality of life in good health) for only 3 weeks to 3 months would yield a very low QALY score. So the service would be said to provide only a very small benefit in terms of QALYs, and thus would be likely to be costly in comparison to the benefit gained.

The concept of the QALY, which depends on a concept of global quality of life and its 'measurement', is here to stay. The cost per QALY is used in the UK by the NICE in judging which treatments the NHS should fund and which it should not fund. Even if the QALY itself were abandoned in the future, some global assessment of outcomes in terms of quality of life is likely to be attempted. It seems there is an unshakeable commitment to attempting to measure the unmeasureable.

We would argue that the best way forward, for the purposes of equitable distribution of health care resources devoted to palliative care, would be the abandonment of quality of life as the goal of palliative care. Qualitative studies on the separate domains, with presentation of results in descriptive terms, should be accepted as the most valid and applicable data that can be achieved for those domains which are not amenable to numerical measurement. Health care providers and administrators, with input from the public, should then use this information to make the difficult but inescapable choices required in resource allocation.

These choices must be made in the context of the demographic changes in the population which have recently occurred and which are predicted in the future. Expensive life-prolonging treatments have been funded in wealthy Western nations for several decades. But as a larger proportion of the population lives into old age and an increasing number develop the incurable and terminal illnesses associated with ageing, more resources will be required simply to provide assistance with the activities of their daily living, and for symptom control. No one could dispute that resources must be provided to ensure basic nursing care and adequate pain control at the end of life. But the implementation of the palliative care philosophy, as described in the WHO definition, is much more resource intensive, and as such it should certainly compete for funding with treatments such as joint replacements, life-prolonging treatments such as chemotherapy, and even curative surgery.

This view is expressed by Maynard in the *OTPM* as follows: 'Increasingly, palliative care managers, both clinical and non clinical, will be challenged and purchasers will demand evidence that the investment in services offered to the dying are more cost-effective than competing interventions such as new drugs approved by NICE, as well as procedures such as hip replacements, coronary artery bypass grafts and renal (a)nalysis [i.e. dialysis]'.[20] He later indicates that society might 'weight' QALYs differently to reflect 'higher social valuation' for care of the dying as opposed to hernia repair.[21] He remains committed to the use of the QALY as a mechanism of allocating resources to the area of palliative care, and thus to the idea of direct comparison of such services with life-prolonging treatments and with procedures such as hernia repair and hip replacement which will provide benefit for some patients.

One obvious problem with this argument is that he seems to be implying that one might have the option of offering no services to the dying. But in the wealthy western nations to which he must be referring, it is unlikely that it would be considered morally acceptable to withhold symptom control and essential basic nursing care plus adequate explanation to patients about the possible treatment options. This basic level of care will surely be regarded as morally obligatory. As Nathan Cherry says: 'It is widely held that terminally ill patients have a right to adequate relief of uncontrolled suffering'. He goes on to point out that this right is recognized by the WHO and medical academies world wide. As he says: 'The corollary of this right is the responsibility of care givers to ensure that adequate provisions are made for relief'.[22]

No one will question the right of suffering patients to receive pain relief. But what is open for debate is whether that pain relief is better and is more cost-effectively delivered by specialist palliative care than by non-specialist care. Of course, it may be the case that for those patients with particularly difficult or complex symptom control problems, specialist palliative care is both more effective and more cost-effective. But what is much more dubious is whether attaching psychosocial and spiritual care and bereavement care is either effective or cost-effective. If the model of palliative care as defined in the WHO philosophy statement is to be extended to all terminally ill patients, then the additional cost in terms of finance and manpower must be justifiable and affordable.

Another obvious problem with Maynard's approach is that since *all* patients will ultimately die, and for the majority of them there will be a period of terminal illness, it simply would not be morally acceptable to society to deny the great majority of people basic symptom control and nursing care when terminally ill. In contrast, a minority of patients would actually ever benefit from a hernia repair or hip replacement.

The macro-allocation judgements that a community makes and the policies it follows reflect the relative values attributed by that community to the three major types of benefits gained from health care. Those relative values also tell us something about the attitudes of members of society to those vulnerable people who are dependent on others for care, or who are terminally ill. Perhaps they also tell us something about attitudes towards death and the degree of acceptance of our inescapable human mortality. It is possible that by influencing and altering macro-allocation policies those responsible for making them may be able to influence society's attitudes to vulnerable people, and perhaps also towards death itself. Thus it can be argued that macro-allocation strategies can be a force for either good or evil.

We have already noted that the WHO ultimately recommends 'simple measures', which we find indistinguishable from competent conventional care. This position is easily justifiable in terms of resource allocation since it does not (at first sight) entail expenditure of resources significantly in excess of non-specialist care. We therefore strongly agree with the WHO's ultimate recommendations of simple measures.

8.3 Conclusions

1 In concluding this discussion of macro-allocation, with particular reference to specialist palliative care, we are suggesting that competent non-specialist conventional care, as ultimately recommended by the WHO, should be available to everyone. Advice regarding symptom control should be available to all health care professionals by education and telephone consultation.

2 Patients whose symptoms are particularly difficult to control, or who have complex care requirements, should be treated by specialist palliative care teams if, but only if, it has been shown that such specialist services can provide more benefit than conventional care for the patients' problems.

3 Macro-allocation cannot be based on the QALY, but requires judgement about the relative benefits of treatment and care packages, about the characteristics of the population, and the use of relevant moral principles.

4 Resources should not be committed for specialist palliative care for everyone until and unless there is clear evidence of benefit over and above conventional care. Qualitative evidence may suffice.

References

1 **WHO** (2004). *Palliative care: the solid facts.* WHO, Geneva: p. 15.

2 **Maynard, A.** (2004). Economics-based palliative medicine. In: *Oxford textbook of palliative medicine,* 3rd edn, ed. D. Doyle, G. Hanks, N. Cherny, *et al.* Oxford University Press, Oxford: p. 50.

3 **Smith, R.** (1999). Stumbling into rationing. *BMJ,* **319**: 936.

4 **Maynard, A.** (2004). op. cit. p. 50.

5 **WHO** (2004). op. cit. p. 16.

6 **WHO** (2004). op. cit. p. 14.

7 **Maynard, A.** (2004). op. cit. p. 49.

8 **WHO** (2004). op. cit. p. 9.

9 **WHO** (2004). op. cit. p. 15.

10 **Beauchamp, T.L. and Childress, J.F.** (1994). Justice. In: *Principles of biomedical ethics,* 4th edn. Oxford University Press, Oxford: p. 330.

11 **WHO** (2004). op. cit. p. 17.

12 **WHO** (2004). op. cit. p. 29.

13 **WHO** (2004). op. cit. p. 30.

14 **WHO** (2004). op. cit. p. 30.

15 **Reinhardt, U.E.** (1966). Rationing health care. In: *Strategic choices for a changing health care system*, ed. S. Altman. Health Administration Press, London: p. 71.

16 **McQuay, H.J., Moore, A., and Wiffen, P.** (2004). The principles of evidence-based medicine. In: *OTPM* op. cit. p. 120.

17 **WHO** (2004). op. cit. p. 15.

18 **Salisbury, C., Bosanquet, N., Wilkinson, E.K.** *et al.* (1999). The impact of different models of specialist palliative care on patients' quality of life: a systematic literature review. *Palliative Medicine*, 13: 3–17.

19 **WHO** (2004). op. cit. p.19.

20 **Maynard, A.** (2004). op. cit. p. 47.

21 **Maynard, A.** (2004). op. cit. p. 50.

22 **Cherry, N.** (2004). The problem of suffering. In: *OTPM* op. cit. p. 8.

Part 3

Critique and reconstruction: some suggestions for a better way

9

Critique and reconstruction: some suggestions for a better way

Introduction

The discussion in the preceding eight chapters was intended to bring out the main weaknesses of the philosophy of palliative care, as it is summarized in the WHO definition and explanation. At the same time the immense strength of the palliative care approach and its benefits for patients have been stressed. In this way we hope to have carried out the main aims of the book: to offer a critique of palliative care (in Kant's sense of establishing its strengths and weaknesses), and to suggest ways in which the palliative care approach might be simplified and reconstructed to provide the basis of good patient care. We have argued that this can be done while still retaining the essence of palliative care as originally described by Dame Cicely Saunders. In this final chapter we aim: to bring together the positive suggestions from the preceding chapters; to develop some of the suggestions; to show how palliative care can enhance other specialties; and finally to suggest a short philosophy statement of our own which avoids some of the weaknesses in the WHO statement. For convenience, and because what we have to say has emerged from argument and a critique of assumptions, we shall continue to call our suggestions a philosophy. Whether it is perhaps over-optimistic to dignify these with that title is not a question which need detain us. We shall begin by examining the credentials of palliative care to be regarded as a specialty.

9.1 Palliative care as a specialty

In order for a branch of health care to be accepted as a specialty it must satisfy three criteria: it must occupy its own distinctive area of practice; it must have its own knowledge base; and it must have an associated skills base.

The area of practice of palliative medicine is the care of dying patients. At present it is most concerned with the care of patients with cancer and motor neurone disease. As we have seen, however, consideration is now being given in the UK to broadening the area to cover other illnesses. The knowledge base of palliative medicine is most obviously that of symptom control, and here there does seem to be a distinctive knowledge base. The skills base is much more controversial. Unlike other specialties, where various procedures and interventions are carried out, specialists in palliative medicine do not themselves carry out any significant procedures, and certainly none of a specialist nature. If there are any skills in palliative medicine they are certainly not hands-on ones. It is unusual in not having a recognizable hands-on skills base. We are assuming that communication skills and counselling skills, even if they can be truly regarded as particular professional skills, are not confined to palliative care.

If then we take into account the defined area of practice around the care of the dying, and the knowledge base of symptom control, palliative medicine just about satisfies the necessary criteria for a specialty. Let us give it a score of 2 or 2.5 out of 3.

Is there any other way in which palliative medicine differs from other specialties? Whether it is different or not palliative care certainly thinks it is. In the words of Michael Kearney, it is not just another specialty.[1] As we have extensively discussed, palliative care has considered it necessary to define its special role via a philosophy statement, the WHO definition of palliative care. This definition describes what palliative practitioners are apparently able to achieve, which is certainly different from what other doctors and nurses are able to achieve. Note that there are no comparable statements about the goals of cardiology, neurology, or orthopaedics.

The definition and its coda emphasize the ability of professionals involved in palliative care to change aspects of the lives of patients and their families which lie far outside the usual remit of health care as delivered by other specialties. We might summarize these points by saying that palliative care aspires to provide holistic or whole person care, or indeed whole family care. This is an important respect in which palliative care differs from other specialties.

What does it mean to provide holistic care? This claim goes beyond giving patients information sensitively, offering competent symptom control, and respecting patients' rights to consent or to refuse the treatment on offer. It goes beyond patient-centred care, which means acknowledging the patients' goals and values. Palliative medicine claims to alleviate emotional, psychological, social, and spiritual suffering, in addition to physical symptoms. There is no other specialty which claims to do all these.

Moreover, palliative medicine claims to be able to alleviate all these forms of distress and improve quality of life, even in the context of dying. Dying is generally perceived to be associated with great distress, yet in palliative care it is held that we can apparently still achieve relief of symptoms, including those of a psychosocial and spiritual nature.

In Chapters 1, 2 and 7 we have criticized what we call the Hippocratic interpretation of holistic care, the attempt to turn it into a technique with the outward trappings of objectivity. What we have tried to suggest is that this Hippocratic interpretation of holistic care is attempting to base it on complex techniques (of dubious validity) when what is needed from professionals is a simple expression of their humanity through quiet listening and friendly reassurance. We have referred to this latter practice as the Asklepian approach to holistic care. What we now want to take up is the question of how to develop this Asklepian model of holistic care, and how to combine it with the Hippocratic approach to physical care.

9.2 The Asklepian model of holistic care

It will be remembered from Chapter 1 (Section 1.2, p. 7) that the temples of Asklepius were said to be populated with harmless serpents whose hypnotic gaze was healing. Healing came from within and occurred when patients accepted their state. This sloughing off of the old skin of false beliefs gave rise to emotional acceptance and spiritual renewal. How can the ideas in this myth be expressed in terms of contemporary health care? How can the ideas be integrated with the equally valid ideas of the Hippocratic tradition? How can the palliative approach as a whole be integrated with the rest of health care? To these questions we shall now turn.

There are two elements which make up what we are calling the Asklepian approach. They are: the attention of the attending physician or nurse, and the inner acceptance or emotional and spiritual peace of the patient.

9.2.1 Asklepian attention

There have been numerous models of the doctor-patient relationship, all of which contain valid points. Firstly, there is a scientific model; a patient can be seen as a 'case' with a diagnosis and a set of symptoms. Secondly, there is the choice model; a patient can be seen as a consumer who makes determinative choices. This consumer view of health care is encouraged by political parties and endorsed by palliative care, which strongly emphasizes the importance of patient choice at the end of life. Thirdly, there is the contractual model; a patient has rights and a doctor has duties. Fourthly, there is the humanistic model; a patient is a person. A satisfactory account of the doctor-patient relationship must attempt to incorporate some of the insights of all these models. We shall shortly show how this might be done, but initially we must identify and describe what might be called Asklepian attention to an individual patient.

One way of identifying this kind of attention is to take the example of the attention we give to a painting, or even that of the attention which an artist might give to a person or landscape, or (as we shall see) to a tree the artist was about to paint. As some readers will be aware, the *Journal of the American Medical Association* (*JAMA*) publishes prints of paintings on its front cover. M. Therese Southgate, who was Deputy Editor of *JAMA*, writes about the relevance of painting to the practice of medicine. In her Preface to *The art of JAMA* she writes of her belief that deep affinities exist between medicine and the visual arts. She goes on to suggest what some of these are:

> Firstly, they do share a common goal: the goal of completing what nature has not. Each is an attempt to reach the ideal, to complete what is incomplete, to restore what is lost. Secondly, the practitioners of each have something in common. The first is observation, keen observation. Even more important than the first because it determines the quality of the first, is the necessity of attention [...] Attention does not seek anything, nor does it impose itself on what is before it. It simply waits in a state of readiness to receive; what it receives is the truth of the object before it. In the end, both art and medicine are about seeing: one looks first with the eyes of the body, next considers with the eye of the mind, and finally, if one has been attentive enough, one begins to see with the eye of the soul. If we remain in this vision, are patient enough and still enough, we begin to hear as well, somewhere deep in the depths beyond where words are formed [...] It is in this same wordless language of the human spirit that the physician sees not just a disease nor even a patient but the person. It is in that moment that healing begins. Paradoxically, the healer is healed as well. That perhaps is the art of medicine.[2]

The above passage brings out eloquently that it is not the feelings of the professional which are important—we have already questioned the familiar doctrines of empathy—but the concentrated attention. Just as the artist tries to see things as they are and ignores her feelings (if any) so the palliative care professional should concentrate on the patient for what the patient is—a unique individual.

Perhaps an analogy from a different kind of art might reinforce the point we wish to make. A musician giving a performance must concentrate on, give full attention to, the music. A successful performance may evoke emotions in an audience, but the performer must remain in control of whatever feelings he or she may have, otherwise he or she might lose their place! The attention, the listening with both the physical ear and the inner ear, takes precedence over any emotion. In a similar way, the attending physician or nurse directs their gaze towards the patient, and is totally receptive to what the patient is communicating. This way of learning what the patient needs is both more effective and more humane than imposing structured interviews from the outside. It is in terms of this analogy from art that we are interpreting the Asklepian notion of the healer's hypnotic gaze.

9.2.2 Asklepian attention and Hippocratic observation

Granted this interpretation of the Asklepian notion of attention the question might be raised about the extent to which it can be integrated with the interventionist tradition of Hippocrates. The Greeks followed both traditions concurrently. Patients would go to physicians, who, in the Greek world, were considered craftsmen who followed the Hippocratic tradition of rational treatment. The skills of the Hippocratic physicians were practised, but if these failed to bring healing the patient would follow the Asklepian method and instead seek healing in a temple. The physicians of the Hippocratic tradition respected and welcomed the Asklepian tradition with the result that patients benefited from both approaches to healing.

As we have argued throughout this volume the Hippocratic tradition has the upper hand in modern health care. Evidence-based medicine is dominant in all spheres and doctors are increasingly encouraged and exhorted to follow protocols and patient pathways. Palliative care has embraced this culture too. This is no doubt a good thing, but in palliative care it has been taken too far and the attempt is being made to create an objective science of emotional and spiritual care. This we hold to be a serious error. Palliative care must retain the Asklepian tradition, which stresses the attention we must give to each patient with his or her story. There is no science or social science which can substitute for this. Palliative care professionals must not hide their human gaze behind questionnaires, counselling, or quality of life scales. 'Tools' may mend the car but not the broken spirit!

The public more widely also seem to want aspects of the Asklepian tradition. When modern orthodox medicine has failed to cure them they frequently seek alternative therapies or means of healing, which commonly are not evidence-based. It is interesting that alternative medicine stresses the patient's role in his or her own healing. Whether we like it or not, patients seem to want to retain the key elements of the Asklepian ideal, alongside modern orthodox medicine.

Palliative care is, and ought to remain, different from other specialties by retaining the Asklepian ideal of healing through focusing on the patient before us. It must resist a total take-over by the over-zealous interpretation of that ideal in terms of the Hippocratic tradition, a protocol-driven process which risks treating all similar diseases, and all biologically similar patients, in the same way. In this respect, palliative medicine must not become just another specialty. But how are the two traditions to be combined? Can we unify the insights of both traditions?

Dame Cicely Saunders was clear that this ought to be done. In *Watch with me* she writes: 'I think the one word "watch" says many things on many different levels . . . it demands respect for the patient and very close attention to his distress. It means really looking at him, learning what this kind of pain is like, what these symptoms are like, and from this knowledge finding out how best to relieve them'.[3] In this description we can identify both Hippocratic and Asklepian attention.

The same point is made in a very different way by Martin Buber. The twentieth century philosopher/theologian introduced a new phrase into the language. In his most famous book he speaks of the 'I-Thou' relationship.[4] Buber contrasts that relationship with what he calls the 'I-It' relationship. In the I-It relationship we see an object, or perhaps another person, in terms of causality or function. Most obviously we are in an I-It relationship with a thing we make use of for some practical purpose, a hairbrush, say. We can also be in an I-It relationship with another human being. This is not necessarily a bad thing; we all must make use of each other if social life is to continue. But we are in an I-Thou relationship with a friend, if we appreciate each other for what we are, and questions of instrumentality are not in the forefront of our minds. The question Buber raises is whether it is possible to combine the two attitudes. This is precisely the question we are raising when we ask whether we can combine the Asklepian mode of attention with that of the scientific mode of Hippocrates. He discusses the question in terms of a striking image:

> I consider a tree. I can look on it as a picture; still column in a shock of light, or splash of green shot with the delicate blue and silver of the background. I can perceive it as movement; flowing vein or clinging pith, suck of the roots, breathing of the leaves, ceaseless commerce with earth and air and the obscure growth itself. I can classify it in a species and study it as a type in its structure and mode of life. I can subdue its actual presence and form so sternly that I recognize it only as an expression of law, of the laws in accordance with which the component substances mingle and separate. I can dissipate it and perpetuate it in number, in pure numerical relation. In all this the tree remains my object, occupies space and time, and has its nature and constitution. It can, however, also come about, if I have both will and grace, that in considering the tree I become bound up in relation to it. The tree is now no longer It. I have been seized by the power of exclusiveness. To effect this it is not necessary for me to give up any of the ways in which I consider the tree. There is nothing from which I would have to turn my eyes away in order to see, and no knowledge that I would have to forget. Rather is everything, picture and movement, species and types, law and number, indivisibly united in this event. If I face a human being as my Thou, and say the primary word I-Thou to him, he is not a thing among things, and does not consist of things [...] nor is he a nature able to be experienced and described, a loose bundle of named qualities. But with no neighbour and whole in himself, he is Thou and fills the heavens.[5]

This passage is both obscure and inspiring. The details of its meaning can be passed over, since for our present purposes it is making four main points. Firstly, it is stressing the importance of accurate observation, and observation with a variety of dimensions concerned with type, number, law, composition, forces in opposition, and so on. If we apply the analogy to the context of health care we can interpret it as saying that there is no substitute for a careful and accurate diagnosis of the patient's symptoms and underlying disease, and this (Hippocratic) concern must take priority. Secondly, this (Hippocratic) kind of observation can change into a particular kind of attention directed specifically at this object or person. 'I become bound up in relation to it [...] I have been seized by the power of exclusiveness'. This is the Asklepian moment. Thirdly, the observation and the particular kind of attention are compatible: 'to effect [this attention] it is not necessary for me to give up any of the ways in which I consider the tree'. Fourthly, this kind of attention is at the same time a recognition of the value of this unique individual—'If I face a human being as my Thou [...] he is not a thing among things [...]'.

In short, Buber is saying via this example that the I-It and the I-Thou relationships can be unified. In our terminology, the Hippocratic, scientific, observation of symptoms is compatible with Asklepian attention to the unique value of the patient we are attending. This is the point which Dame Cicely Saunders is making when she unpacks the meaning of the term 'watch' in the passage quoted above.

There is one further question which must be answered. We are maintaining that the Hippocratic or scientific attitude is compatible with the special attention of the Asklepian attitude. But how can both exist at the same time? How can a patient at one and the same time be observed with a scientific attitude and be given the special attention of the Asklepian attitude? The answer is that there seems to be a problem here only if we think of the situation in terms of a misleading image. If we interpret the attentive gaze of the physician or nurse as being like that of a searchlight which is either on or off then we might think that there was a problem. But a better image (to continue with lighting) is with the varied and coloured lighting of a disco. Human beings are capable of switching among a range of technical attitudes and a number of human attitudes. It is this facility which makes it possible for the professional-patient relationship to be both technical and human, or Hippocratic and Asklepian. But this is difficult to achieve – it requires experience and maturity.

9.3 Asklepian acceptance and spirituality

We said that there are two main elements which make up the Asklepian approach—the special kind of attention, and the inner healing or making whole which comes from an acceptance of one's mortality. We have discussed the first of these and must now turn to the second. How can the ideas of an inner peace and acceptance be encouraged among patients?

In discussing this question we are returning to issues of emotional and spiritual care raised in Chapter 7 and elsewhere. We are also going back to questions raised in Chapter 1, Section 1.7 (p. 13) but not so far addressed. What do we think are the answers, or the approaches to answers, raised by the ultimate questions posed by the philosophy of palliative care? As we said in Chapter 1, the palliative care approach assumes but does not make explicit a set of assumptions about good ways to live and to die. Can we be bold enough to try to make explicit some answers to, or at least some way of looking at, these ultimate questions? What is it that makes life worthwhile or gives it significance or meaning?

Most people at some time ask themselves questions such as the following. What does my life add up to? Have I ever done anything really worthwhile? In the last phase of life people might ask themselves questions with more urgency. These questions must be distinguished from equally natural questions about the mode or processes of dying. Questions of the latter sort are Hippocratic questions which, however important, we shall not address here. Questions of the former sort concern what it is that makes life of significance and gives meaning to it.

In the WHO philosophy statement the term 'spiritual' rather than the term 'religious' is used regarding these ultimate questions. The reason for this is that while the origins of palliative care were in religious orders contemporary professionals wish to appeal to a much wider constituency. They therefore use the word 'spiritual' since it covers the wider issues. Now, questions of this spiritual nature, concerning the meaningful life, admit of answers of two different sorts. The first we can deal with reasonably easily, but the second is much harder.

The first set of questions is the one which arises when spirituality takes a religious form. Many people still have religious beliefs. Even if the beliefs have lain dormant for many years they may well come back to the surface in the last phase of life. The responsibility for dealing with or offering comfort and reassurance to such patients really rests with the chaplain or other religious authority. For those who sincerely hold a religious belief, what gives their life meaning is something which comes from outside them. What is important to stress here is that for such patients their lives are *given* meaning; they can see their lives as part of a larger framework. The task of their spiritual adviser, in the sense of their religious adviser, is then to offer comfort by trying to reinforce their beliefs in the overall framework. However difficult this may sometimes be in practical terms there is no theoretical problem about the aim.

Since most palliative care units or hospices have their own religious advisors palliative care professionals need not be mainly involved here.

However, other people do not have such beliefs. For them their lives are not given meaning from the outside. Spiritual meaning must therefore be found in the way their lives are lived and ended. What are the factors which make a life seem meaningful? This raises the second and more complex set of issues. The issues are partly conceptual: certain factors make a life count as meaningful. Someone whose main activities are gambling and spending the proceeds on himself might have an exciting or enjoyable life, but it hardly counts as a meaningful life. The factors are partly empirical or experiential: the adoption of certain purposes causes people to feel that their lives are meaningful. For example, someone who trains for and obtains a job may feel that his life is meaningful, and experiences like falling in love or sharing an interest with a friend can also cause us to feel that our lives are meaningful. The factors are partly moral: for we morally approve of the meaningful life and withhold the term 'meaningful' from lives which lack certain purposes or qualities. An embezzler might be very skilful, but we would not call his life meaningful.

Granted the acceptability of this three-aspect analysis we are left with the question of what can be said to patients in the final phase of their lives if they seek reassurance about these anxieties when facing death. Note, of course, that by no means all patients do wish such reassurance, or, if they do, wish to receive it from palliative care professionals. It would be quite wrong to imply to patients, whatever the motivation, that relief of physical symptoms is in any way tied to discussion of these possible end of life worries. But for those patients who do wish such discussion there is some general advice from Dame Cicely Saunders already quoted: people are not in a specialist palliative care unit to die but to live until they die.[6] Our questions, then, are: What are the purposes, the activities, the conversations which would count as a meaningful end to a life, which would cause or enable someone to feel that their life has ended in a meaningful or worthwhile way, which would be morally good, and which would enable them to 'live until they die'?

It is obvious, but perhaps should be stated, that to be meaningful is not the same as to be profound or socially important. Ordinary activities and relationships are what are likely to constitute a meaningful end to a life, especially when the person is already very sick. Hence, our suggestions may be obvious or banal, but again it may be worth stressing that professionals should not try to be over-ambitious. There is a tendency to assume that bad relationships must be put right at the end of life but this may not be possible for a variety of reasons, and perhaps it is a mistake to encourage attempts which may fail. Again, the idea of a good death or a meaningful end may be more in the minds of palliative care professionals than patients. Nevertheless, a few points should be made.

First of all, visits from friends and relatives are to be encouraged—the dog too if there is one. It is common for patients to want a shopping trip and a final return home may enable a patient to say goodbye to familiar surroundings. Of course, the family may resist this, and in this kind of context the WHO philosophy has created a problem by giving the relatives' wishes a priority equal to that of the patient.

Some hospices or palliative units have an artist or writer in residence, and for some patients the consciousness that life is coming to an end can spark off creative ability which has lain dormant for a lifetime.[7] It is through the arts that some patients can express what they find it difficult to say, others again may wish to contribute to research. Many palliative care professionals are protective of their patients and resist attempts to have them enrolled in trials. Nevertheless, some patients may wish to take part in trials as a way of taking part in a morally good project. As we have said, the purposes and activities of the meaningful life must be morally acceptable.

These simple activities can be said to comprise the final fulfilment of a human life. J.S. Mill, in analysing what self-development consists of, argues that we all have what he calls a 'distinctive endowment'. The qualities which make up that distinctive endowment are: 'the human faculties of perception, judgement, discriminative feeling, mental activity, and even moral preference which are exercised only in making choice'.[8] Now many of the simple purposes and activities which we have mentioned can be seen to fall into Mill's list, but arguably the most important, and as Mill suggests, the one which is common to all of them, is the ability to make a choice. The consciousness that, however sick one is, one retains some marginal control over one's life, is an important factor which can make the end of a life seem worthwhile.

The ability to exercise some marginal control over one's life, to exercise some choice, is often depicted as important to the idea of human dignity, as we have seen. It is therefore highly desirable that where possible a patient at the end of their life should be given some room for choice. But we are emphatically not going down the path of many, perhaps the vast majority of those in health care ethics, who make choice an essential factor for human dignity.[9] The idea of informed, rational choice, of consent and refusal of treatment, is of course important in health care ethics, and we have stressed this, but it is not essential for human dignity; it is just one of the ways in which dignity can be shown. Even when there are no choices possible human dignity can be shown in an acceptance of the inevitable. Human dignity can be shown, and in palliative care often is shown, in courage, humour, and concern for others;

this is central to the Asklepian philosophy. The poet Andrew Marvell, in describing the execution of Charles I, portrays the dignity of the King:

> He nothing common did, or mean,
> Upon that memorable scene;
> ....
> But bowed his comely head
> Down, as upon a bed.[10]

9.4 Honest hope

We have suggested some simple ways in which palliative care professionals have a role to play in enabling patients to feel that their remaining weeks are worthwhile (quite apart from the Hippocratic task of symptom control). The results of a recent study indicate that patients want two things from their carers: accurate information, and hope.[11] The trouble is, as the writers of the article and many of those taking part in the study realize, it is difficult to combine the two in all circumstances. As the Editor of the *BMJ* puts it: '[M]any patients want to be told but do not want to know'.[12] Patients can pick up when the truth is being fudged and therefore feel patronized, but equally they feel discouraged and demoralized if the information is given too bluntly or insensitively. How are hope and truth-telling related in palliative care? We shall begin by analysing the concept of hope.

What does it mean to hope that something will come about? Hope has two essential elements. The first is that the object of hope must be desired by the hoper—for example, a patient may desire the prolongation of life or the relief of suffering. The second element is that the hoper must believe that the fulfilment of hope falls within a range of probabilities. At one extreme, it is clear that one does not hope for something that one already knows will happen. At the other, one must believe that the object of hope is at least possible: obviously one cannot hope to live to 100 years old if one is terminally ill at 50. Hope requires that the object of hope falls within a range of physical probabilities which excludes the certain or the merely logically possible, but includes the unlikely. Whilst one may wish for that which is merely logically possible, one cannot hope for it.

As an aid to understanding the significance of hope the image of a rope is illuminating in two ways. Firstly, a rope has strands twisted together against each other. In the case of hope one strand is the positive anticipation, the other is the fear that what you hope for might not happen—for instance going home from hospital. Secondly, a rope can be something we hold on to, a vision of the future. It is part of our nature, our identity as persons, that we have a concept of time, and having this concept of time, and of time passing, we constantly look to the future. Indeed, we gaze so constantly towards the future that the quality of our existence now is highly dependent on how our future looks to us. If we are not able to hope for good things in the future, the quality of our present existence is much impaired.

Thus, if there seems nothing to hope for, we start to feel hopeless. Now hopelessness is associated not just with the absence of pleasure, but rather with a particular wretchedness and misery. Hopelessness is not just a cause of suffering, it is itself a state of suffering. If we are depressed then everything seems hopeless, and hopelessness is the cause of very much suffering in a depressive illness. It is also true however that it is possible to experience hopelessness without being depressed, at least in any clinical sense. Nevertheless, if one feels unable to sustain hope for very important goods in life one is likely to become depressed.

What are the links between hope and truthful communication in palliative care? The answer to this question raises issues of ethics. Our roles as doctors, nurses, or other health professionals entail our making certain choices about what we will say, and how we will act towards patients, their families, and each other.

We can consider first the choices we make about what to say. What we say, especially the information we give, will influence what others around us are able to hope for, the way they see the future. The most obvious example of this in palliative care is the information we choose to give to patients and their families. For it is this information which serves as the basis for their hope. We tell them what is possible, and often give them information about the probabilities of future events. In this way we often exert significant influence over what patients are able to hope for.

But since it is they who hope, because it is they who determine what they desire, and they who ultimately judge its probability, it is the patients themselves who are the origin and the enduring source of that hope, not us. So whilst in choosing what to say we can and do influence their hopes we must remember that the hope is theirs, not ours. Whilst we ought to encourage people to hope for outcomes which are probable, and to help them adjust away from hopes for the extremely unlikely, at the same time we ought not to seek to control their hopes. There is a fine line between the two! On the other hand, if we misinform them, so that they believe that something good may happen to them when that is actually extraordinarily unlikely, then we have given them the basis for a false hope.

Now some relatives suggest that it is better to have a false hope than to be in a state of hopelessness, and some professionals go along with this. The professionals' motivation is that false hope is better than hopelessness. On the other hand, there is a general moral obligation to tell the truth. Whatever special circumstances may lead to a breach of this obligation such as a conflict with another moral obligation, for example to keep a promise, the general force of the obligation to tell the truth is not disputed in any culture. Three reasons are usually given for this. Firstly, if we are to maintain meaningful communication with each other the truth must be told. Individuals, institutions, or politicians who do not habitually tell the truth, or who spin it in misleading ways, are in the end simply disbelieved, even when the news is good. Secondly, the truth must be told if people in general are to be able to make their own rational choices about their futures. Thirdly, it is not thought to be respectful of a person to give misleading information, even to protect them from unpleasant or wounding truths. None of us, of course, wants to hear bad news, but that is compatible with saying that we ought to be given the truth. To be over-protective is to be patronizing and paternalistic. For at least these three reasons ordinary morality condemns the telling of lies in everyday life.

Against this it might be argued that we do allow a breach of the truth-telling rule in circumstances where there is a strong counter obligation; we mentioned above the counter obligation of promise keeping. Now it might be argued that another counter obligation is to prevent the state of hopelessness, and if we can do this by giving false information then there is an obligation to do so which overrides the general obligation to tell the truth. Is it morally justifiable to give false information in order to engender a false hope if the motivation is to prevent the establishment of that state of misery which is hopelessness? Many relatives, and perhaps some professionals, think that it is.

But there are three moral arguments in opposition to this justification. The first is that the patient is likely to discover that the hope is false, so will lose the hope anyway. The outcome is then likely to be hopelessness coupled with resentment. Moreover, the trust which is central to a good relationship with a patient will be eroded. This is bad not only for a specific relationship but is likely to cast a shadow over palliative care more generally; palliative care professionals will gain the reputation of not telling the truth or of distorting it with spin. The second reason is that the issue of the patient making inappropriate choices on the basis of misleading information remains unresolved. The third reason is that the problem of having deliberately deceived the patient by giving false information remains. Telling a lie is still wrong no matter what the motivation behind it.

Professional guidance does not usually include a direct prohibition on creating false hopes, but indirectly it does. The relevant guidance pertains to consent. Doctors in particular are clearly instructed to describe the benefits of proposed treatment, but they must also disclose serious or frequently occurring risks. By implication therefore they are instructed not to give false information which may form the basis of false hope.

Yet, despite these conclusions from ordinary morality and professional guidance, patients are sometimes given excessively optimistic information about the potential life-prolonging benefits of treatment. They then form false hopes. For example, we recently met with the case of a patient with rapidly progressive motor neurone disease and a high likelihood of respiratory failure within a few weeks. The neurologist concerned prescribed Riluzole with the stated aim of prolonging life. In reality the neurologist did not believe this would come about, and prescribed this expensive drug merely in order to give the patient hope. The result was that the patient hoped for many months of life and planned his life around this false hope.

It could be argued that in this case, even if one were prepared to prescribe this expensive drug when one believes there is almost no prospect of benefit, one ought to explain the low likelihood of benefit to the patient, who is then able to develop his hopes based on correct information. In general then, in terms of information about the prognosis of diseases and the potential benefits of treatment, ordinary morality and professional guidance indicate that we ought to tell the truth and we ought not to give incorrect information, even if our motive is to encourage a false hope and so avoid hopelessness. Our role is to give patients a truthful portrayal of the probabilities, from which they can generate their own hopes.

It is worth noting in passing that what we have offered as a discussion of the concept of hope can apply also to the concept of futility.[13] The argument here seems to be that even if a treatment is futile from the physiological point of view it might have psychological benefit. In our terminology, this is saying that it can be a good thing to engender false hope. The argument really amounts to saying that if a patient believes, or can be encouraged to believe, that a treatment is of benefit it should be given. But firstly, this is surely advocating a return to the practice of a bygone age when coloured water was prescribed as a placebo. Secondly, it is paternalistic to assume that a patient cannot face up to the truth, that for him or her there is no treatment which will have a life-prolonging outcome. Thirdly, the morally wrong nature of the practice is compounded if it is carried out simply because the relatives insist on it.

In palliative care there are other aspects of treatment and care which are not concerned with the prolongation of life. These are treatments and care which may diminish suffering. Information on these may provide the basis for patients' hopes, but here again there is a need for caution. We should note once again that the WHO definition makes claims about improving the quality of life of patients and their families, and about the impeccable or faultless treatment of pain and physical and psychosocial and spiritual problems. In the context of our discussion of hope the ethical issue with this definition is that it may be giving patients a false hope regarding what palliative care can do for them and their families. Do we really believe we will always achieve an improvement in patients' and families' quality of life, and will our management of all distress be 'impeccable'?

In discussing hope we must not forget the professionals themselves who work in palliative care. Those who constantly work with and care for patients who are going to die require some enduring hope at the deep centre of their own being. Hopelessness is as destructive for the professional as it is for the patient. For some, and this of course is the origin of palliative care, it will be a religious hope. Others will have a hope based on a belief in the fundamental good in human beings, or a belief that life is worth living and meaningful to the end. We shall develop this point in the next section.

It should also be noted that the wider beliefs and personality of the palliative care professionals will affect how they are perceived by patients. A recent study of doctors' communication with patients with breast cancer indicated that patients valued a 'relationship' with the doctor—they wanted to see each other as individuals: 'The perception of being regarded as an individual was communicated in several ways. Non-verbal cues included eye contact, smiling and touching. The simplest verbal strategy was for the patient to be told she was special. The most common strategy was brief conversation unrelated to disease'.[14] The ability to do this requires the doctor or nurse not just to have Hippocratic or technical skills but to be a particular kind of person. The importance of being a particular kind of person, which we have touched on in several previous contexts, is one which we shall now discuss further. The particular type of person in one guise is the 'friendly professional' discussed in Chapter 7, Section 7.2, and in another the challenger of orthodoxy mentioned on p. 3. In our terminology the 'particular type of person' is the Asklepian doctor. The problem for medical education is how to combine the two essential aspects of the good health care professional—the Hippocratic and the Asklepian.

9.5 Personal and professional development

As a preliminary it should be noted that many philosophers and perhaps most medical educators would argue that the question of the doctor's personality, however important, is not a matter of ethics. For the majority of contemporary philosophers the function of morality or ethics is to provide a system of checks and balances which enable us to live in harmonious and co-operative relationships with each other. In short, duties are always to other people and never to yourself.

But these views are quite recent. Historically speaking there have been many accounts of the nature of morality which give a large role to becoming a particular kind of person. The Greeks for instance stress this, and there is a strand in Christian thought which stresses that the Kingdom of Heaven is within you, and the problems of the moral life are depicted as those encountered on a pilgrimage. Even Kant, whose maxim of respect for persons as ends is often quoted, is rarely quoted in full. In full, he says: 'Respect human nature, whether in your own person or in that of another'.[15] In other words, he is stressing that we have duties to ourselves, to our human natures. As far as medical education goes, studies such as the one discussed above on patients' reactions to doctors treating patients with breast cancer, bring out that, as J.S. Mill says: 'It is important not only what men do, but also what manner of men they are that do it'.[16] Whether we regard this as making it a matter of morality or not is something for philosophers to discuss. It is certainly important. The immediate task then is to discuss some issues of personal and professional development.

We can begin by noting that medical and nurse educators are aware of the importance of what is variously called personal and professional development, or continuing medical education. Broadly speaking, we might say that the reason for this emphasis in medical education at all levels is an awareness on the part of medical educationists that doctors and nurses must not only be up-to-date with the latest scientific information, but must also be able to think for themselves, or to have minds of their own, to enable them to translate the many and conflicting claims of evidence-based medicine and government initiatives into humane treatment for individual patients.

Yet there is an important ambiguity in the idea of having a mind of one's own which can distort programmes of personal and professional development, and health care education more generally. The ambiguity can be brought out if we distinguish two different ideas which might be implied by having a mind of your own: independence of mind and individuality of mind.[17] Independence of mind is shown in the kind of support or justification which a person might offer for a belief. In more detail, independent minded persons can exhibit three qualities.

Firstly, their beliefs, medical or otherwise, are based on evidence or argument. This sweeping statement must of course be qualified and developed. Different types of evidence are needed in difference sorts of situation, and sometimes, if the matter is very technical, we ourselves may not be able to state the evidence, and may need to rely on the word of experts. But even here we may be able to assess whether the person really is an expert in that field, or whether the 'evidence' is really just ideology or pharmaceutical hard-selling.

Secondly, independent-mindedness requires an ability to understand what we claim to have in our minds. For example, suppose someone is told that the structure of the DNA molecule consists of a double-helix. How does that person make this statement their own? The claim would need to be understood in several different senses. Thus the person would need to understand some concepts of biochemistry and of mathematics and how they might be linked, and also the wider context and significance of the claim. Understanding here is something we can have more or less of, and to the extent that we have it we are more or less independent-minded.

Thirdly, we are independent-minded if we are critical of the evidence or argument for a belief. For example, we may come to hold that the evidence for a proposed treatment is insufficient, or of the wrong kind, or that the side-effects or the cost of the treatment have not been mentioned. Critical appraisal of appropriate evidence is indeed one of the characteristics common to any academic discipline, and typically goes on at lunchtime meetings in hospitals and postgraduate centres.

From the above brief account of what it means to be independent-minded it will be clear that in the context of healthcare the person of independent mind has the (excellent) characteristics which belong to what we have called the Hippocratic approach. Let us turn now to individuality of mind.

Individuality of mind concerns differences in the content of people's beliefs, rather than in the rational basis or evidence for their beliefs. It concerns their imaginations, their intuitive abilities and their sensitivity. The beliefs of an independent mind purport to be well-founded, whereas those of a mind with individuality purport to be distinctive, unusual, original, challenging, idiosyncratic, imaginative, intuitive or sensitive. Individuality can be shown in many ways: for example, it may be shown in an unusual direction of interest. The person with the individual mind may know about unusual or less commonly known things, and this can be shown as much in the sciences or medicine as in the arts. Again, individuality of mind can be shown in a great depth of knowledge in some areas. This kind of specialized knowledge is often dismissed by saying 'He knows more and more about less and less'. But a highly specialized direction of knowledge and skills is desirable in medicine and other areas. As a gesture towards allowing individuality of mind to develop the medical curriculum in the UK now allows Special Study Modules (SSMs) in which students can follow their interests in science, medicine, or the humanities through short periods of in-depth study which may lie in unusual directions of interest.

A third aspect of individuality of mind can be shown in a variety of ways. Perhaps it is best expressed by the term 'lateral thinking', a term which was introduced by a former lecturer in medicine at the University of Oxford, Edward de Bono.[18] The main point made by de Bono is that we tend to see the world, including the areas of it which constitute our professional lives, in terms of certain patterns or groupings. But these are only some of the many possible patterns or groupings. The person with a disposition to lateral thinking is the person who can break away from the familiar patterns and suggest new ways of looking as things, or non-routine ways of behaving. Intellectually, lateral thinking may emerge as a sceptical disposition towards received opinion and ways of doing things.

Lateral thinking of the kind relevant to individuality of mind is illustrated in the philosopher Wittgenstein's anecdote about the fly in the bottle.[19] The fly buzzes against the glass and cannot escape, but there is no stopper in the bottle; if the fly changes direction it can escape. The person of individual mind who can think laterally can show the fly the way out of the bottle! Another way of putting this might be to say that the person who can think laterally is the one who shows imagination and can enable us to see the world, including the world of healthcare, in fresh ways. Standard evidence-based treatments are no doubt usually the best, but they may not be the best for this particular patient. Individuality of mind enables us to develop the ability praised by David Roy 'to think thoughts others dared not imagine' (see Chapter 1, p. 3).

What are the connections between independence of mind and individuality of mind, and personal and professional development or continuing medical education? The classic text which guides us here is J.S. Mill's essay *On Liberty*.[20] We have already quoted from Chapter 3 of this essay, in which Mill tells us that the end of man is the highest and most harmonious development of his powers to a complete and consistent whole (p. 208). These powers are developed by pursuing ends which are rich and complex and therefore suitable for bringing out the potentialities within us. In more detail, Mill argues that we all have what he calls a distinctive human endowment, which can be developed. As we have already seen, the qualities which he thinks make up this endowment are: the human faculties of perception, judgement, discriminative feeling, mental activity, and even moral preference which are exercised only in making a choice.[21] We might say that these qualities are distinctive of what can be called the generic human self. These qualities, Mill holds, can be developed, and it is encumbent on us as human beings to develop them. It is our claim that developing this endowment and developing independence of mind are one and the same, and are one essential component in personal and professional development.

Individuality of mind by contrast is concerned with the development of at least some of those qualities and interests which are peculiar to a given person. However the development of those idiosyncratic qualities will make use of the generic features of the human endowment, the features on Mill's list, but will turn them in a direction unique to a given individual person. Mill argues for this in a second and complementary strand in his thinking. When the second strand is uppermost he stresses the importance of the conscious and choiceful pursuit of objectives which express authentically one's own uniqueness as a person. According to this strand in his thought, it is important to be oneself as opposed to conforming to custom. A custom may be a good one, he says, but 'to conform to custom merely as custom does not educate or develop [in a person] any of the qualities which are the distinctive endowment of a human being'.[22]

Independence of mind and individuality of mind will both find their ultimate justification in self-development (or personal and professional development), but in different ways: independence of mind leads to the development of our distinctively human endowment, the generic aspects of the self, whereas individuality of mind leads to the development of our personal uniqueness, our individuality, the idiosyncratic aspects of the self. These two aspects of development are necessary and sufficient for total self-development. One aspect can be seen as the Hippocratic side to health professionals, and the other the Asklepian side.

Now it is reasonably clear in general how independence of mind can be developed in the health care professions. The process will be one of reading journals, attending courses on the latest treatments and the basic science behind them, and above all learning to exercise ones critical abilities. This is the Hippocratic side to medical education.

The development of individuality of mind represents the Asklepian side to medical education and it is much harder to achieve. In many ways it is discouraged, and certainly what we might term the ethos, the climate in which health care professionals operate, is not friendly to individuality of mind. Consider, for instance, the sameness of presentations with their overhead slides and power point presentations. Indeed, it is not unamusing that at a time when educationalists are emphasizing the importance of communication and listening skills, the professionals themselves seem unable to give or follow a talk without constant visual aids! The result is a dreary sameness. The teachers or clinicians one remembers are the ones with the individual or even the eccentric approach; they enrich one's imagination as well as developing one's knowledge. Anecdotes and enthusiasms are more memorable than bullet points, just as watching and listening are more therapeutic than harassment with assessment tools! The Asklepian side to patient care is important and must be re-stated and cherished in health care.

One important way in which individuality of mind can be cultivated is via the arts and humanities. This is being increasingly recognized in health care education circles. As we have previously noted, most medical schools now have Special Study Modules (SSMs) which can include some study of the arts and humanities. In the context of our argument this kind of study has many merits.[23] For example, literature deals above all with qualitative distinctions. There is no one scale on which the actions and interactions of the characters in a novel or play can be measured. One event or action is not just a different quantity of another; rather novels, plays, and films deal with the qualitative richness of human interaction and the possibilities of tragedy involved. The kind of understanding which comes from this is quite different from that produced by science or social science. Science and social science search for patterns or laws, but these are always abstractions from the complex realities of actual events and actions. Descriptions of the 'role of the patient', or of the 'stages of bereavement' do not describe the behaviour or feelings of any actual person. The insight they provide is abstracted from the complex motivation and interrelatedness of actual patients.

It must be remembered, of course, that while the arts and humanities are important vehicles for the cultivation of individuality not everyone responds well to them. But everyone can have their own life outside their profession. Indeed, it may be worth stressing that as far as relating to individual patients is concerned, the experience of friendship or of having an interest or hobby outside the clinic may be more relevant to patient care than attending a course on managing bereavement or how to measure the quality of life. This belief lies behind our stress on the 'friendly professional'.

9.6 **Teams**

So far, in this expansion of our views on how palliative care must evolve, we have been assuming a one-to-one relationship between patient and professional. But of course in all areas of health care the importance of teams is stressed. What are teams and how do they fit in to the philosophy of palliative care? We have already discussed this at some length in *Palliative care ethics*[24] but will approach the issues here from a slightly different point of view. This is worth doing since the WHO definition does mention teams, and if the palliative care approach is to be adopted more widely then some attention must be given to teams, teamwork, and their problems.

What are teams? Definitions can prematurely point thinking in the wrong direction. For example, the management idea of a team may not be helpful as a model for a medical team. There is some guidance from the origins of the word—teams consisted of oxen or horses pulling together for a common purpose. Out of this simple idea of a team ploughing we can take some points.

Firstly, a team involves a group; one horse is too few, and ten is too many. The right number depends on the second characteristic of teams: teams have a common aim, and the right number in the team will depend on the aim. Thirdly, someone in the team carries overall responsibility for the decisions of the team. Team meetings and interdisciplinary discussion are important, but teams in health care are not a democracy. The team leader, usually a consultant, would be foolish not to listen and to take very seriously the views of those who have most contact with a given patient, but in the end it is the consultant who carries legal responsibility for the team decision on matters of medical treatment. Fourthly, teams must have some way of evaluating their success. Note that we said 'evaluating' and not measuring. To speak of measuring is to suggest numbers (usually misleading) and to play into the hands of politicians and chief executives. The success of a major football team might be measured in terms of the number of matches won, goals scored and so on. But to use this approach to East End Juniors would be quite inappropriate. For this team you might want to evaluate its success in terms of the skills learned, the physical exercise, and the comradeship. These cannot be measured in any numerical way.

The fourth point is clearly important for teams in palliative care. The presence of specialist palliative care in-patient units in general hospitals might be deplored by managers, because the death of terminally ill patients in the general hospital, rather than in an independent hospice, nursing home or community hospital, will elevate the mortality figures of the general hospital and thus lower its place in a league table. But counting deaths in palliative care is a very poor way of evaluating the success of the team. The quality of care in a patient's final weeks is much more relevant, but this is something which cannot be put on a numerical scale. It will be remembered that we have argued against the acceptability of such scales (Chapter 2, Section 2.2, pp. 35–42).

Properly functioning teams are important therefore in the evolution of palliative care, and we refer readers to *Palliative care ethics* for a fuller discussion of the nature of teams, their merits and their problems.

9.7 The desirability of a philosophy of palliative care

In this final chapter we have so far dealt with some issues not previously discussed in our critique, and we have developed other points already mentioned. We are now in the position where we shall try to pull the argument together. After all, it might be said, if we offer a critique of palliative care and the WHO philosophy it is only fair that we state our alternative position. On the other hand, granted our critique of the philosophy of palliative care, it might be argued that a philosophy is just a distraction from the real business of actual care. Is a philosophy of palliative care really desirable?

We think that it is desirable to describe and use a philosophy of palliative care, for several reasons. Firstly, there is the fashion for mission statements, philosophy statements, and so on. If a single officially recognized statement is not formulated, each palliative care team is likely to draw up, display, and attempt to live by, its own individual philosophy or mission statement. But a measure of conformity of approach is desirable so that patients and the public know what to expect from their treatment. Secondly, the word 'palliative' is not universally understood, and patients and the public do not know what palliative care is, so a philosophy statement is necessary in order to inform them of the aims and nature of such care. Thirdly, it is important to produce a new philosophy statement which will influence the care and treatment of terminally ill patients for the better, and which avoids, as far as possible, the problems and adverse consequences inherent in the present WHO statement.

If we assume that these reasons point to the desirability of attempting to formulate a philosophy we can move on to consider the question of the possibility of such a philosophy. In brief and general terms, what would the new philosophy statement say? It would need to satisfy certain criteria.

Firstly, the aims, values, and assumptions described in the statement should be consistent with the aims, values, and assumptions of health care in general. Secondly, these aims should be consistent with professional codes and the law. It is essential that a new philosophy should not influence health care practitioners to act contrary to their professional codes or the law. Thirdly, the aims and values of palliative care should not cause its practitioners to pursue goals which are unattainable or inequitable in terms of the resources of a publicly funded health care system.

Granted the acceptability of these criteria we propose the following brief account of a philosophy of palliative care. It is intended to avoid the pitfalls we have identified in the existing philosophy, but to preserve the essence of palliative care as it is currently practised. We shall first draw together the positive conclusions we have reached about how palliative care should evolve, and then summarize our view with a brief philosophy statement which encapsulates our entire position.

9.8 Towards a new philosophy

We maintain that the central aspect of palliative care is symptom control delivered humanely with adequate information. Much of our thinking on this has been influenced by our view that the philosophy of palliative care should be consistent with health care ethics in general and should form an integral part of the latter. Granted that, we argued that the WHO statement that palliative care 'intends neither to hasten nor to prolong death' should be rejected because of its intrinsic ambiguities. Health care practitioners may justifiably hasten death as a foreseen but not intended effect of treatment whose aim is the relief of pain and distress at the end of life. In such cases the benefit of symptom relief outweighs the harm of bringing an inevitable death nearer. On the other hand, prolonging life is a goal of health care, and is often appropriate in the palliative care context. Guidance for practitioners on these matters should state that the benefits, harms and risks of a treatment in the patient's particular circumstances should be weighed up carefully. This includes analysing as far as possible the illness scenarios and ways of dying which are likely to occur with and without the treatments.

In the philosophy of palliative care, as in health care ethics and the law generally, letting die must be permitted. Letting die here means withholding or withdrawing a life-prolonging treatment when its harms and risks exceed its benefits. Health care practitioners who act in this way neither cause nor intend to cause the patient's death. This point is frequently misunderstood and misrepresented. It is simply a confusion to say that the patient has been killed by the doctor[25] when a treatment is withdrawn because it is not only doing no good but is actually causing harm to the patients (and the family) by prolonging the period of dying.

This point is sufficiently important to be worth developing. There is a significant moral difference between intentionally causing the death of a patient by administering lethal medication (mercy-killing or euthanasia), and withholding or withdrawing a life-prolonging treatment because of lack of net benefit with the result that the patient dies of the underlying illness (letting die). The philosophy of palliative care, health care ethics, and law, must continue to uphold the prohibition against killing which protects all members of society. In law, professional codes and clinical practice, it is necessary to distinguishing between intentional acts which cause the death of patients (acts described as killing or euthanasia) and the withholding or withdrawing of life-prolonging treatment so that the illness causes death (acts regarded as letting die).

We have argued that clinicians can be guided by advance statements or living wills towards the kind of treatments which an incompetent patient might wish (if the clinician thought it appropriate) and the kinds of treatment which such a patient might refuse. Patients should therefore be encouraged to think about these matters in good time. There is an education task here for the public and professionals.

We also argue that there is a good deal of confusion around 'Do not attempt to resuscitate' (DNAR) decisions. It is not generally realized either that attempts have a very poor chance of success in palliative care, and that they are associated with considerable harms, such as broken ribs and an undignified death. Moreover, when we are dealing with patients at the very end of their lives it is not at all clear what the justification could be for attempting to resuscitate a patient who will very shortly die of the underlying disease process.

In discussing these matters we have argued that the doctrine of double effect is too complex to use in clinical practice. What is needed is general guidance involving a clear drawing of the distinctions between killing and letting die. The importance of observing valid and applicable advance refusals of treatment must also be stressed. Individual cases can be very complex of course and principles and points of view may appear to conflict. But just as we expect a good clinician to identify complex medical symptoms, classify them, reach a diagnosis, and propose a management plan, or we expect a judge to follow similar procedures of analysis and legal classification in complex legal cases, so it should be possible for a health care professional to identify the moral issues, classify them, and so reach an ethically sound decision. As we said in Chapter 1, this is called the method of casuistry, and as a method it is similar to that used in medical diagnosis and treatment decisions and in law.

Turning now to the WHO statement as it affects relatives, we argued that whereas a special relationship, founded on an implicit promise and associated with special obligations, exists between professionals and patients, there is no special relationship, and no implicit promise, between professionals and the relatives of patients. Improvement in the quality of life of the relatives of patients should not be an aim of palliative care. Moreover, pursuing the interests of relatives at the expense of the patient's interest cannot be justified in any health care setting including palliative care; achieving a benefit for the relatives cannot justify inflicting harm on the patient. Relatives should be given information necessary for the care of the patient, and such further information as the patient wishes to be disclosed. But whereas caring for relatives is not an intrinsic aim of palliative care, professionals should be ready to offer friendly advice.

Quality of life is one of the most frequently used concepts in discussions of health care. The trouble is that it is also frequently used in many other contexts, including popular discussions. The result is that, whereas it is usually clear in a given context what the phrase means, there is no constant meaning even in health care. It is therefore not surprising that the attempts to turn it into a technical term in health care inevitably fail. This is apparent from the many failed attempts to construct a quality of life scale.

Quality of life is (unsurprisingly) essentially qualitative and evaluative and cannot (logically) be rendered quantitative. Apart from the inevitable failure of attempts to devise scales there are moral issues involved in using quantitative questionnaires and structured interviews. Patients who are in the last phase of life should not have these questions imposed on them. We therefore draw the conclusion that quality of life is a concept which should be dropped from the technical vocabulary of palliative care; the hazards, moral and intellectual, of attempting to devise or use such scales far exceed any benefit to patients. Whereas attempts to measure quality of life as a global concept are bound to fail there is a place for qualitative studies of given aspects of palliative care. Indeed, and this we have argued in the context of resource allocation, it requires to be established that specialist palliative care, as described in the WHO definition, is actually better for patients in all respects than more conventional end of life care. Qualitative studies would be informative here.

We noted that the WHO philosophy statement stressed the importance of the 'impeccable' assessment and treatment of the patient's emotional, psychosocial, and spiritual state. But it is often forgotten that this is an intervention like any other, and the consent of the patient must be obtained for any such intervention. Professionals in palliative care are often so convinced of the benefits of this aspect of their approach that they forget it might be harmful to some patients, that it should never be tied to the control of physical symptoms, and that it is certainly an intrusion on privacy. The patient's consent is therefore required.

Going along with this aspect of the palliative care approach is the belief that a close personal relationship between patient and professional is desirable. We have serious doubts about the desirability of a close personal relationship between patient and professional in any branch of health care, including palliative care. On the other hand, we are equally opposed to the detachment of the client-counsellor relationship, so often advocated in palliative care. What is essential from the professional is sensitive explanation and advice based on experience. These are especially effective if delivered by a 'friendly professional'.

As far as spirituality is concerned, some patients may not wish such matters to be raised; others may wish the advice of a chaplain; while others again may find ultimate meaning in simple activities, in the arts, or in the company of their friends. Neither assessment nor intervention should be forced upon them for their own spiritual good. Indeed, the idea of a spirituality scale is comic in its absurdity.

We have offered several types of reason for our criticism of the undue emphasis which palliative care specialists have placed on attending to families, and prioritizing their quality of life and psychosocial problems. One of these reasons is that such attention is demanding of resources which we think might be better devoted to a wider population of patients. This point is of particular importance in the UK where the government wishes the palliative care approach to be extended to the care of all patients. The problem of macro-allocation arises here. Resources should not be devoted to attempts to implement the WHO philosophy unless there is clear evidence of benefit over conventional end of life care. Such evidence is of course hard to obtain, but qualitative evidence would suffice.

Micro-allocation is of course inevitable; judgements have to be made regarding patients' ability to benefit from specialist care. Competent non-specialist palliative care ought to be provided and, going along with that, telephone advice by specialists should be available to all health care professionals; and specialist palliative care professionals should attempt to spread their expertise to others by educational programmes. The result would be that specialist palliative care could then be concentrated on those patients whose symptoms are difficult to control or whose care requirements can be met only by a specialist team. On these points we find ourselves in agreement with the UK NICE *Guidance on supportive and palliative care for adults with cancer 2004.*[26]

9.9 A new philosophy statement

This account of our views can now be condensed into a final statement which we believe is realistic in terms of what palliative care can achieve and what it should represent, if its philosophy is to be adopted by other branches of health care.

Palliative care is the care of patients whose disease is incurable and is expected to cause death within the foreseeable future. The aims of treatment are to minimize pain and other symptoms, and to prolong life, but with a minimum of burdens and risks as assessed by individual patients and professionals working together. The informed consent of competent patients regarding treatment is sought by presenting information honestly but sensitively. Refusal of treatment is respected.

Incompetent patients are treated in accordance with their best interests as judged by the health team following examination of the medical circumstances and exploration with the family of what can be known of the patient's wishes. In deciding the best interests of the patient, the team will respect valid advance refusals of treatment and will as far as possible interpret any statement of the patient's values and wishes in terms of possible treatment decisions. Professionals provide support to patients:

- By ascertaining how much information patients seek and providing it sensitively;
- By listening to patients' views about their own goals and values;
- By discussing the possible impact of various treatments on their lives so as to work out which treatment will most benefit a particular patient;
- By providing advice based on experience.
- Explanation, professional advice and encouragement are given to caring relatives within the limits necessitated by the rules of confidentiality towards patients.

We wish to suggest in conclusion that our proposed philosophy of palliative care has several merits:

1 **Realism.** We do not claim that palliative care can diagnose and treat every problem, physical, emotional, social, and spiritual, of terminally ill patients, far less those of their families, and far less 'impeccably'.

2 **Fairness.** We do claim that priority in care should be directed at patients, not at patients and families equally; that specialist palliative care should be available only to those patients whose symptoms cannot be controlled in conventional end of life care settings; that telephone advice on specialist care and educational programmes should be available to all health care professionals.

3 **Humanity.** We argue that very ill patients should not be subjected to questionnaires, intrusive interviews and numerical measurements of dubious validity. Instead, they should be supported by a professional who has current Hippocratic expertise in matters of symptom relief, has the attentive gaze of the Asklepian physician, but can also engage in friendly conversation on the wider issues of life.

4 **Adoptability.** We argue that more modestly and realistically stated the palliative care approach has something to offer other specialties. It reminds them that in the present frenzied political and more general cultural ethos of 'fighting disease', 'meeting targets' and 'saving lives', the essence of the quiet art[27] may be lost.

References

1 **Kearney, M.** (1992). Palliative medicine – just another specialty? *Palliative Medicine*, 6: 39–46.
2 **Southgate, M. T.** (1997). *The art of JAMA.* Mosby, St Louis, MO: p. xii.
3 **Saunders, C.** (2003). *Watch with me.* Mortal Press, Sheffield: pp. 1–2.
4 **Buber, M.** [1923] (1937). *I and thou*, translated by R.G. Smith. T & T Clark, Edinburgh: p. 3.
5 **Buber, M.** [1923] (1937). op. cit. pp. 7–8.
6 **Saunders, C.** (2003). op. cit. p. 46.

7 **Kirklin, D.** (2004). The role of the humanities in palliative medicine. In: *Oxford textbook of palliative medicine*, 3rd edn, ed. D. Doyle, G. Hanks, N. Cherny, *et al.* Oxford University Press, Oxford: pp. 1182–9.

8 **Mill, J. S.** [1853] (1962). *On Liberty.* Collins, London: p. 187.

9 **Downie, J.** (2004). Unilateral withholding and withdrawal of potentially life-sustaining treatment: a violation of dignity under the law of Canada. *Journal of Palliative Care,* **20**(3): 143–9.

10 **Marvell, A.** [1650] (1972). An Horatian Ode upon Cromwell's Return from Ireland. In: *The new Oxford book of English verse,* ed. H. Gardner. Clarendon Press, Oxford: pp. 329–33.

11 **Kirk, P., Kirk, I., and Kristjanson, J.** (2004). What do patients receiving palliative care for cancer and their families want to be told? A Canadian and Australian qualitative study. *British Medical Journal,* **328**: 1343–6.

12 **Smith, R.** (2004). Medicine and man's fall. *British Medical Journal,* **328**: Editor's choice.

13 **Zucker, M. B. and Zucker, H. D.** (ed.) (1997). *Medical futility.* Cambridge University Press, Cambridge.

14 **Wright, E. B., Holcombe, C., and Salmon, P.** (2004). Doctors' communication of trust, care, and respect in breast cancer: a qualitative study. *British Medical Journal,* **328**: 864–7.

15 **Kant, I.** [1785] (1948). *Groundwork of the metaphysic of morals,* translated by H.J. Paton. Hutchinson's University Library, London: p. 96.

16 **Mill, J. S.** [1853] (1962). op. cit. p. 188.

17 **Downie, R. S.** (2004). Personal and professional development: a mind of one's own. *Clinical Medicine,* **4**: 332–5.

18 **deBono, E.** (1990). *Lateral thinking.* Penguin Books, London.

19 **Wittgenstein, L.** (1953). *Philosophical investigations.* Blackwell, Oxford: para. 309.

20 **Mill, J. S.** [1853] (1962). op. cit.: p. 186.

21 **Mill, J. S.** [1853] (1962). op. cit.: p. 187.

22 **Mill, J. S.** [1853] (1962). op. cit.: p. 187.

23 **Downie, R. S. and Macnaughton, R. J.** (2004). *Clinical judgement: evidence in practice.* Oxford University Press, Oxford: pp. 153–196.

24 **Randall, F. and Downie, R.S.** (1999). *Palliative care ethics,* 2nd edn. Oxford University Press, Oxford: pp. 79–102.

25 **Randall, F.** (1997). Why causing death is not necessarily morally equivalent to allowing to die—a response to Ferguson. *Journal of Medical Ethics,* **23**: 373–6.

26 **NICE** (2004). *Guidance on supportive and palliative care in adults with cancer.* National Institute for Clinical Excellence, London: Section 9.

27 **Virgil** [29–19 B.C.] (1956). *Aeneid,* translated by W.F. Jackson Knight. Penguin, Harmondsworth: 12, 397.

Author Index

General Index

Note to index: the term "versus" (*vs*) is used for "as compared with"